PLANT-BASED
DIET
IN 30 DAYS

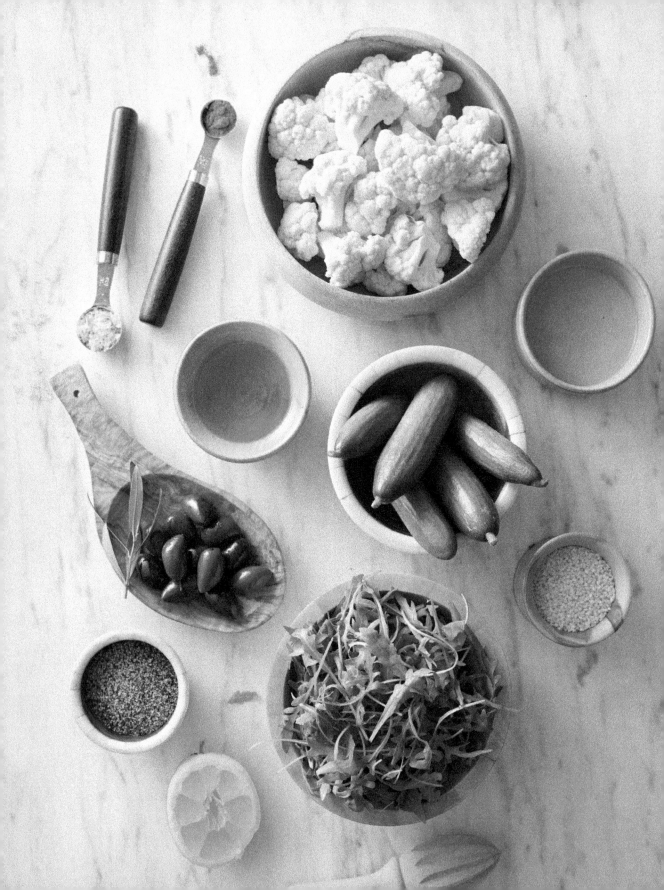

PLANT-BASED DIET IN 30 DAYS

A Cookbook and Meal Plan for an Easy Transition to the Plant-Based Diet

SARA TERCERO

Photography by Darren Muir

ROCKRIDGE PRESS

Interior and Cover Designer: Amanda Kirk
Art Producer: Janice Ackerman
Editor: Gleni Bartels
Production Manager: Holly Haydash
Production Editor: Jenna Dutton

Photography © 2021 Darren Muir. Food styling by Yolanda Muir.
Author photo courtesy of Photo by Erb/Dufault Photography.

Cover: Sweet Potato, Kale, and Red Cabbage Salad with Creamy Avocado-Lime Dressing, page 85

ISBN: 978-1-64876-833-0 | eBook 978-1-64876-253-6

R0

I DEDICATE THIS BOOK TO MY PRECIOUS FAMILY:

DAVID, MIA, EZRA, AND ALEXA,

WHO MAKE MY STORY UNIQUE AND

GIVE ME PURPOSE.

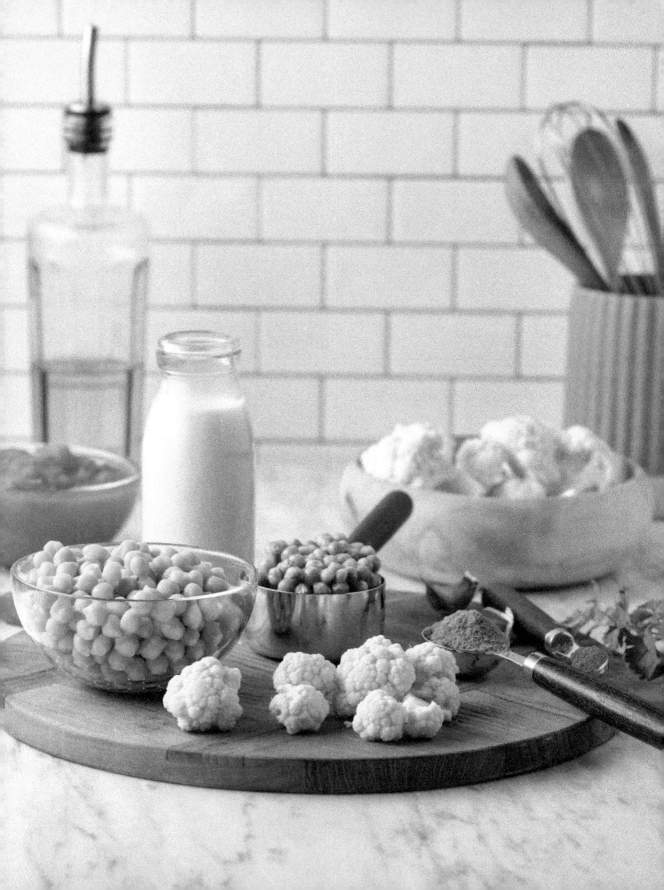

CONTENTS

Chickpea Coconut
Curry, page 114

INTRODUCTION

RESEARCH INDICATES THAT PLANT-BASED DIETS ARE EFFECTIVE AT preventing disease. Chances are, if you are reading this, you are curious about how plant-based eating can help you. Perhaps you have high cholesterol, high blood pressure, or your doctor has warned you about prediabetes or recent weight gain. Maybe you are concerned about the environmental impact and would like to make a change toward a more sustainable future. For whatever reason you are reading, this book provides simple, straightforward information, backed by studies to illustrate the reasons that plant-based eating is your solution. It shares the basics of plant-based nutrition and debunks the myths to pave the way for you to make a successful and fearless transition to a plant-based diet. Once you understand the why, I show you how by giving you the tools, recipes, and shopping lists to begin an easy and delicious 30-day eating plan that anyone can follow. The 100 recipes in the book set you up for success by being easy to cook, tasty, and nutritionally sound, and include tips for cooking, storing, and varying the ingredients to your own personal tastes and abilities.

Before my own transition to a plant-based diet, I struggled with excessive weight gain, vitamin deficiencies, and sluggish energy levels. As a professional chef, I always had abundant food at my fingertips, and reaching for the fastest options often resulted in my overconsumption of high-fat and less nutrient-dense foods. After having three babies back-to-back, many extra pounds, and a thyroid condition, I decided to try eating plant-based for one year to see if all the hype was true. Now I am going into my third year, with no plans to turn back. In fact, I have been so profoundly affected by the change, it has become my mission to help others find an easier path to better health through eating a whole-food and plant-based diet.

I am thrilled to be sharing my simple, no-nonsense approach to plant-based eating with you, whether it becomes your permanent lifestyle change or just a great excuse to eat more delicious plants.

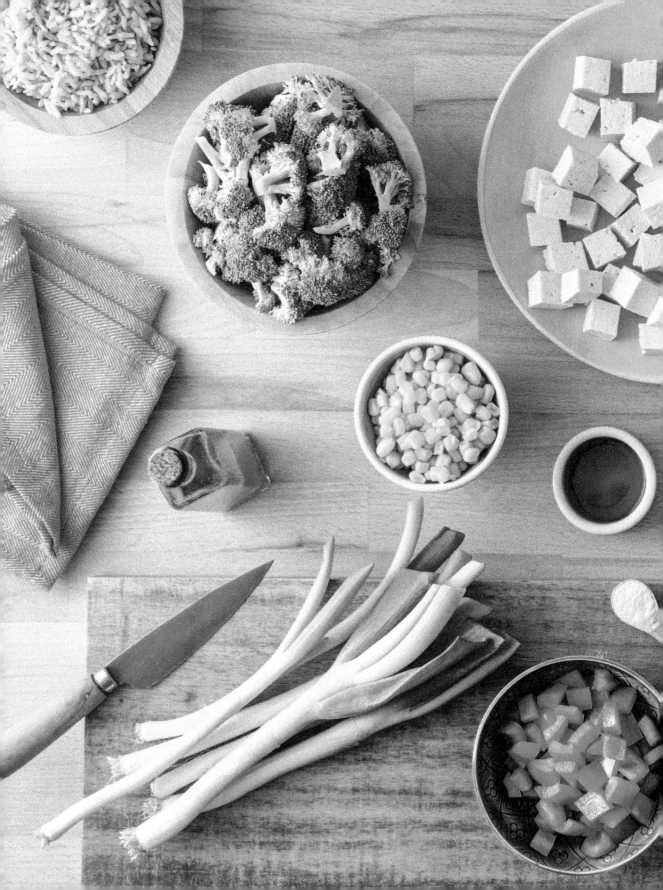

PART 1

THE
PLANT-BASED
DIET PRIMER

Baked Flaxseed-Battered
French Toast, page 132

CHAPTER ONE

WHY GO PLANT-BASED?

WELCOME TO YOUR PLANT-BASED EATING ADVENTURE! My love for plants runs deep, and I'm thrilled to guide you on your journey to increased health and vitality. Thanks for taking this step, which has such enormous potential to transform your life, with me. For those who have centered their meals on animal products their whole lives, the journey to a plant-based diet might seem overwhelming, but with the right tools, anybody can do it. I promise to ease you onto a plant-based path deliciously and seamlessly with 30 days of easy, colorful recipes that will satisfy your hunger and nourish your body.

THE POWER OF PLANTS

I bet you've heard the buzzword "plant-based" thrown around a lot lately. What was once seen as a diet for those on the fringe has now gone mainstream, thanks to documentaries, news reports, and high-profile enthusiasts like celebrities and athletes who all applaud the diet's merits. The jury is in, and the verdict is that eating more plants is good for us. This is not just another fad diet. Plant-based eating has had devotees as far back as biblical times, and many cultures and religions have eaten this way for centuries. Even the Academy of Nutrition and Dietetics states that "well-planned plant-based diets support health and are appropriate throughout all life stages, including pregnancy, lactation, childhood, and adulthood, as well as for athletes."

What We Mean by Plant-Based

There are many definitions of the term "plant-based," but for the purposes of this book, let's define it as a diet that is rich in fruits, vegetables, whole grains, legumes, nuts, and seeds, and void of any animal products, including eggs, dairy, and honey. Here are a few of the main tenets of the plant-based diet you'll follow on this meal plan:

100 percent plants: The recipes included here are all plants, all the time. Some who call themselves plant-based consume animal products in moderation but eat mainly plants, usually an 80/20 split. Although this can be a healthy and reasonable eating pattern, it's important to learn to appreciate the rich diversity of plant-based flavors and textures and get comfortable creating meals using only plant-based ingredients before transitioning to any other long-term dietary plans.

Focused on whole foods: Most people who seek a plant-based revolution in their life do so for health reasons, so abstaining from processed foods like cheese and meat alternatives, which can contain chemicals and additives, is advised. As such, these recipes will focus on whole, minimally processed foods whenever possible. Foods like whole-grain breads and pasta, tofu, and unsweetened plant-based milks are okay in moderation and go a long way in making this lifestyle change sustainable, so they're included in the meal plan, but the majority are whole foods.

Less salt and sugar: The standard American diet is brimming with preservatives and added salt and sugar, which has led to a culture of disease that could be helped by increasing consumption of whole foods and reducing intake of salt and sugar. I use salt sparingly throughout to allow the natural flavors to pop, but you can even omit it altogether if you'd like. When sweeteners are necessary, I choose natural versions like dates and maple syrup, which are less processed.

RELATED LIFESTYLES

As I mentioned before, there are a lot of ways to define a plant-based diet. Add to that the plethora of similar diets, and it can be hard to keep things straight. Below are a few related diets and lifestyles, explained.

Vegetarian and pescatarian: Vegetarians don't eat animal flesh but will consume by-products that come from animals that don't cause harm, including eggs and cheese. Pescatarians follow the same guidelines as vegetarians but also include fish and seafood in their diets. For some, the added versatility of these lifestyles can be less challenging and are often a natural gateway to a fully plant-based diet.

Whole-food, plant-based (WFPB): WFPB refers to a diet where you eat only whole foods in their most unrefined form possible. While it's often synonymous with a "plant-based" diet, many also use this term to describe a more restrictive diet that also eliminates salt, oil, and sugar—sometimes called "SOS-free" eating.

Vegan: Veganism is more of a lifestyle choice than a dietary one. It focuses on the ethics of cruelty, which translates into avoiding all products that exploit any animals in any way. In addition to not eating meat, dairy, seafood, or any other animal by-products, vegans won't wear clothing made from animals, including leather and furs, or use products that include animal by-products or that have been tested on animals. This also includes exploitation of "human animals" who are suffering oppression or exploitation in any form, as veganism is understood to be an intersectional route of political activism.

How Plants Can Change Your Life

The benefits of transitioning to a plant-based diet are bountiful. Here are a few ways choosing plants can change your life:

Put you in a better mood: According to research by the Physicians Committee for Responsible Medicine, eating animal products causes inflammation in the body, which in turn may trigger or worsen anxiety and depression. Since plant foods are naturally high in antioxidants, which lower inflammation, people may see a boost in their mood on a plant-based diet. Also, since animal foods are higher in fat and protein, they require more energy to digest, which can leave you feeling sluggish and fatigued.

Save you money: Meat, dairy, and processed foods tend to have a higher price tag than plant-based whole foods. I was astonished at how many groceries I could buy on my food budget when I switched to a plant-based way of eating, and I'm sure you will be, too.

Manage your weight: A plant-based diet may help you lose weight. Many studies have been done on this subject. In a study conducted by the University of South Carolina of five different diets over six months, those on the vegan diet lost more weight than those who were omnivorous. For a more personal anecdote, I lost 15 pounds in my first year of plant-based eating without restricting calories.

Keep your heart healthy: Plant-based foods are low in fat and cholesterol so they're a great choice to keep your heart healthy. Studies have shown eating plant-based not only prevents heart disease but can reverse its effects and reduce the risk of developing heart failure up to 42 percent.

Lower your risk of disease: People who eat a diet high in fruits and vegetables are at a lower risk for type 2 diabetes than those who don't—by as much as 50 percent! And abstaining from the saturated and trans fats found in dairy products, meats, and other processed foods can help ward off cognitive diseases like dementia and Alzheimer's.

Reduce your carbon footprint: Research suggests that eggs, meat, and dairy have a much higher carbon footprint than plant-based foods. Making the switch can drastically lessen your carbon footprint.

A BALANCED PLATE

When transitioning to a plant-based diet, many people are nervous about cutting out meat because they assume they will be deficient in protein, iron, or essential vitamins like B_{12}. But it's easy to have a balanced plate on a plant-based diet, and I worked hard to keep the dishes and meal plans in this book nutritionally sound. Each recipe will have nutritional information to help you determine which will work best for needs and also to help familiarize you with plant-based nutritional breakdowns. Below we'll dive deeper into just how this balance can be accomplished.

Getting Your Protein Fix

Anyone who has ever followed a vegetarian or plant-based diet has been asked by concerned loved ones, "But where do you get your protein?" As a culture, it seems we are obsessed with protein, but why is protein so important? Proteins are the building blocks your body needs to make and repair your tissues, blood, bones, and hormones, and are described as both "complete" and "incomplete." Complete proteins contain all nine essential amino acids that are vital for protein synthesis, nutrient absorption, and more. There is much speculation whether plant-based complex proteins exist, but soy, quinoa, and buckwheat all fit the bill. And although many plant proteins are incomplete sources of protein, eating a varied diet will ensure that you meet your daily dietary needs (approximately 56 grams of protein for men and 46 grams for women). In most cases, protein deficiencies are very rare and seen only in those who are extremely malnourished. The following chart gives a rundown of the grams of protein in a serving of common plant-based foods.

SOY AND A PLANT-BASED DIET

There's also much discussion on whether soy is a healthy form of protein. Consuming soy in its less processed forms like tofu, tempeh, edamame, and miso is a great way to get your protein fix. The main controversy surrounding soy is about plant estrogens, but many sources agree soy is safe for most people to consume in moderation. However, if you've had breast cancer or thyroid disease, you should consult your doctor before adding soy to your diet, as the estrogen levels could be a concern.

Grams of Protein Per Serving		
FOOD	**STANDARD SERVING SIZE**	**PROTEIN**
Black beans	1 cup	15g
Buckwheat	1 cup	5g
Cashews	¼ cup	4g
Chia seeds	2 tablespoons	4g
Chickpeas	1 cup	15g
Green peas	1 cup	9g
Hemp seeds	3 tablespoons	11g
Lentils	1 cup	18g
Quinoa	1 cup	8g
Tofu	½ cup	10g

Filling Up on Good Carbs

Despite the popularity of low-carb or no-carb diets, there's evidence indicating that carbs are good for you. In fact, they're your body's main source of energy. According to the Mayo Clinic, carbs should make up between 45 and 65 percent of your daily calories (between 225 and 325 grams a day). But there's an important distinction between simple and complex carbs. Complex carbs, like quinoa, oats, and brown rice, are full of fiber, which burns slowly, releasing more energy over a sustained period. Many simple carbs, like processed foods and sweeteners, don't have any nutritional value and are best eaten sparingly. However, some simple carbs are found in fruit and vegetables that are high in fiber, which makes them a great addition to your diet regardless. When developing this meal plan, I considered fiber content and nutrients in conjunction with carbs to ensure that the recipes are devoid of simple sugars and chock-full of healthy, complex carbs and macronutrients found in fruits, vegetables, and whole grains.

Enjoying Healthy Fats

Much like carbohydrates, fats have a bad reputation, but they help with many metabolic processes and increase feelings of fullness. Most sources agree that 20 to 30 percent of your daily calories should come from fats, but they also agree that focusing on the number of fat grams per day matters much less than the quality or type of fat being consumed. Saturated fats and trans fats are typically found in animal products and processed foods and are a leading cause of cardiovascular issues. Some healthy plant-based fat sources include nuts, seeds, avocados, extra-virgin olive oil, and nut butters.

Other Nutrients

Almost every vitamin and mineral need, including iron; folate; calcium; vitamins A, C, D, and E; and omega-3s can be satisfied by a varied plant-based diet. The exception to this is vitamin B_{12}, which is only found in animal products. So how can plant-based eaters get their B_{12}? Many foods, including plant-based milks and whole-grain cereals, have been fortified with the essential vitamin, so just check the labels to make sure you're grabbing a fortified version. To get the daily recommended amount of 2.4 micrograms of B_{12}, you can eat fortified foods two or three times per day, take a low dose (about 10 micrograms) supplement daily or take a higher dose (at least 2,000 micrograms) variety weekly.

If you have any nutrition-related concerns, I encourage you to contact your health-care provider for a checkup and have a conversation about options that are right for you before starting any kind of dietary lifestyle change.

Tofu and Vegetable
Fried Rice, page 161

CHAPTER TWO

PREPARING YOUR PLANT-BASED KITCHEN

NOW THAT WE'VE HAD A PRIMER ON THE BENEFITS OF A PLANT-BASED diet and the importance of balanced eating, let's get into the fun stuff—the food! Plant-based eating is not only about healthy bodies, happy animals, and a better environment; it's also about vibrant flavors and delicious meals. In this chapter, I'll guide you through the process of preparing your kitchen for the next 30 days—and beyond.

A FRESH START

Are you ready for a fresh start? I know it may seem like an enormous undertaking, but we'll start from square one. While we may be purging your space of some old favorites, with the amazing new ingredients and flavors you'll be trying, I'll bet you won't even miss them.

Clean Out Your Kitchen

One of the easiest ways to set yourself up for success is to get rid of any temptation by clearing out any ingredients that don't fit the guidelines including all processed foods, meats, seafood, dairy, eggs, and, yes, even your refrigerator door full of condiments. Many dressings and sauces are packed with preservatives, sugars, and salt. Feel bad about food waste? Donate your nonperishables to a local food bank. See if your neighbors want any of your ingredients with a limited shelf life or freeze them to handle later.

The Foods You'll Be Eating

Now your pantry might look pretty bare, but it won't be for long! Soon it will be full of delicious, nutritious, and really colorful ingredients. Here are a few you can expect to see in the recipes that follow. Most of them will likely be familiar, but you'll be amazed by how versatile they can be.

Fresh fruit and produce: apples, arugula, avocados, bananas, beets, bell peppers, berries, broccoli, butternut squash, cabbage, carrots, cauliflower, eggplant, garlic, ginger, kale, mushrooms, onions, potatoes, spinach, spring lettuce mixes, sweet potatoes, tomatoes, and zucchini

Food for the fridge and freezer: frozen bananas; frozen berries; frozen vegetable blends; plain, unsweetened plant-based yogurts and milks; tempeh; and tofu

Food for the pantry: canned and dried beans and legumes, healthy oils, nuts and seeds, nut butters, whole-grain breads and pastas

INSTEAD OF THIS, EAT THAT

Switching out animal products for plant-based ones is not an exact science, and though there are some pretty good approximations, you'll need to use imagination and ingenuity to find substitutes that will achieve the desired results in a recipe. A beef burger and a veggie burger won't taste the same, but as your taste buds adjust and as you start to enjoy the benefits of a plant-based diet, it will become second nature to reach for these alternatives.

Note that if you are sensitive to monosodium glutamate (MSG), there is a possibility that nutritional yeast can cause an allergic reaction.

NON-PLANT-BASED FOODS	PLANT-BASED ALTERNATIVES
Bacon	Tempeh
Butter for baking	Extra-virgin olive oil, tahini, applesauce
Butter for cooking	Extra-virgin olive oil, avocado oil, coconut oil
Cheese	Nutritional yeast, nuts, tofu
Cheese sauce	Plant-Based Queso Dip (page 139)
Dairy milk	Unsweetened plant-based milks, such as Nut Milk (page 175), Oat Milk (page 176), soy milk, coconut milk, etc.
Egg whites	Aquafaba (the liquid from a can of chickpeas)
Eggs	Tofu, flaxseed "eggs"
Ground beef	Lentils, tofu, walnuts, tempeh
Hamburgers	Veggie burgers, portobello mushrooms
Honey	Maple syrup, Raw Date Paste (page 183)
Shredded meat	Jackfruit, mushrooms
Sour cream	Plain plant-based yogurt, such as almond or soy
Steak	Cauliflower, mushrooms
Tuna or chicken	Chickpeas
Yogurt	Unsweetened plant-based yogurts, such as almond, soy, coconut, etc.

BRINGING THE FLAVOR

This eating plan isn't as restrictive as the whole-food, plant-based diet that also eschews salt, oil, and sugar, but I do take a mindful approach to these ingredients in my recipes. All three are important for developing flavors in a dish, but I'll cook only with heart-healthy oils and unrefined sugars, and salt will always be included in moderation. Below are some of the ingredients I'll use to boost flavors and let the natural goodness of plant-based meals shine.

Healthy oils: Healthy fats help you stay full longer and can add flavor and depth to a dish. Extra-virgin olive oil has zero trans fats and works amazingly for roasting and pan searing. Coconut oil lends a moist texture to baked goods.

Herbs: Fresh and dried herbs add flavor without adding calories or sodium. I especially love to use cilantro, mint, and parsley.

Spices and aromatics: Spices are key in developing plant-based dishes, and I go into more detail on how to stock your spice rack on page 22. Turmeric, curry powder, cinnamon, garlic, and ginger can add depth and heat to dishes.

Sweeteners: I rely on unrefined sugars to sweeten dishes. Dates and maple syrup are easy alternatives to traditional sugars.

KITCHEN EQUIPMENT

In addition to basic utensils like strainers, spatulas, whisks, and tongs, there are a few pieces of essential and nice-to-have equipment.

Must-Haves

A good-quality sharp knife and a cutting board: These recipes will involve quite a bit of chopping and slicing, so I suggest investing in a good-quality chef's knife. A sharp knife also decreases the risk of cutting-related accidents. You'll also want a large cutting board.

Baking dishes: You'll need one 9-by-12-inch oven-safe baking dish for large casseroles and one smaller 8-by-8-inch baking dish.

Blender or food processor: You'll need a high-speed blender, food processor, or immersion blender to make quick work of pureeing creamy soups, as well as chopping hard ingredients like nuts and seeds.

Mixing bowls, measuring cups, and measuring spoons: A standard set of each of these is perfect for all the recipes.

Pots and pans: You'll also need two sheet pans (13-by-18 inches), one large (6-quart) stockpot, one medium (3- to 4-quart) saucepan, and one large (12-inch) skillet. Ideally, they will all be oven-safe versions that can be transferred from the stovetop to the oven, like a Dutch oven or a cast-iron pan.

Nice-to-Haves

Mandoline: These make slicing veggies in uniform sizes quick and easy. They can also come with spiralizer attachments. Always be careful when using a mandoline, as it can easily catch your fingers on the sharp blades.

Nut milk bag: This specialized bag made from fine-mesh netting makes easy work out of straining nut milks. They are inexpensive and well worth buying.

Pressure cooker and/or slow cooker: A pressure cooker, slow cooker, or multicooker is great for batch cooking things like beans and grains.

Salad spinner: A salad spinner can make washing and drying your produce a breeze.

Spiralizer: For dishes with zucchini noodles and the like, you'll want to invest in a spiralizer if you don't want to purchase them premade. You can buy an affordable, handheld one in the produce department of most grocery stores or online.

Wok: The unique shape of a wok makes it a great choice for stir-frying veggies, and its deep bowl is ideal for containing saucy curries.

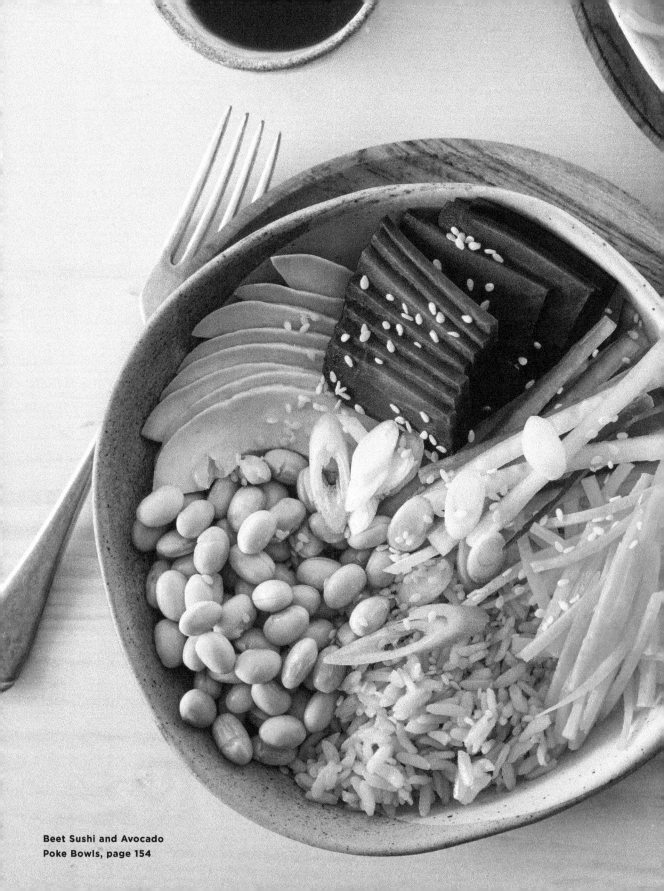

Beet Sushi and Avocado
Poke Bowls, page 154

PART 2

THE
MEAL PLAN
AND RECIPES

Lentil Bolognese,
page 96

CHAPTER THREE

30 DAYS
TO
PLANT-BASED

NOW THAT YOU ARE ARMED WITH NUTRITIONAL KNOWLEDGE and your kitchen is equipped, let's go over the 30-day meal plan. I have designed this plan to set you up for success by making the transition to a plant-based diet smooth and easy. The recipes are tailored to be both simple to execute and tasty. I promise the flavors will get you excited for the next meal and keep your cravings at bay. You can do this! You will be thrilled when your energy level skyrockets and you fall in love with a whole new world of plant-based flavors.

THE 30-DAY PLAN

The plant-based diet is not about deprivation, calorie counting, or weight loss. In fact, although losing pounds is often a perk, we aren't focusing on it at all. Instead, we'll concentrate on enjoying your plate full of colorful and nutritious food. It's a delicious way to satisfy your hunger and improve your health at the same time!

Within days of starting the plan, a few things will become apparent as your body begins to acclimate. You'll notice a shift in your energy level after eating. You'll feel energized and not sluggish like you would feel after eating the same amount of food as your previous diet. Your digestion will improve, leaving you with fewer digestive issues. By the end of the 30 days, you'll likely have shed a couple of pounds and your blood sugar, cholesterol, and blood pressure should be improved.

Remember, you can make a sustainable lifestyle change using this 30-day plan. I'm providing an easy-to-follow blueprint to a happier and healthier you that will be the foundation upon which you build a lifetime of health and vitality.

HOW IT WORKS

The plan is divided into four chapters (one per week) that include menus, shopping lists, and associated recipes—all tailored for simplicity and success. A few things to keep in mind about the plan:

Shopping lists: Each week of the meal plan will feature a comprehensive list of "Ingredients You'll Need" to make all the recipes and a handy "Staples to Check For" section full of ingredients you might already have in your cabinets.

Prep this: This section lets you know when a recipe needs to be started the night before, like Peaches and Cream Overnight Oats (page 82). If a recipe calls for another recipe in the ingredients list, it'll give you the option to prepare them along with the main ones on the menu (but for any "double-recipe" recipes, there is always a store-bought alternative given, just in case).

Serving sizes: The recipes were developed with a serving size of two people in mind, with each recipe yielding two to four servings. For a larger family or bigger yield, simply double or triple the recipe. Or for a smaller yield, scale the recipe in half.

Leftovers: The four-serving recipes are designed to give you leftovers that can be eaten as is or used as part of another dish. Leftovers are a lifesaver when you're meal planning. You can cook once and eat twice!

Snacks: You'll notice that snacks are not included in the meal plan, but some plant-based ideas for keeping the "hangries" at bay are a handful of nuts and berries, plant-based yogurt and granola, smoothies, or vegetable sticks and hummus. All these ingredients are used in the recipes, so they'll be on hand when you need them, or you can pick up some extra fruits like apples, oranges, and bananas.

TIPS FOR SUCCESS

Here are a few tips and tricks that will be intrinsic to your success in transitioning to a plant-based diet and staying on track.

Bowls are your new best friend. A big bowl of ingredients brimming with different textures, colors, and flavors is often a brilliant default meal. You can take leftovers from several different meals and pile them on top of some greens for the ultimate in noshing satisfaction. They prevent food waste, you ingest a variety of nutrients, and they're delicious!

Jump on the meal-prep bandwagon. Meal prep is another tool you'll need in your corner. Choose one or two days a week to batch cook a couple of recipes or prep ingredients so you'll have easy meals at your fingertips. Store meals in individual portions to bring to work or heat up for a quick dinner. Not only is it convenient, but it is also genius for portion control.

Keep it colorful. The first bite of food is taken with the eyes. I believe that if food looks pretty, it tastes better. Plus, the more colors you can add to your meals, the more nutrients you'll get. Each color of the rainbow is associated with being higher in different vitamins. For example, green foods are high in potassium and red foods are loaded with vitamin C. Bulk up your nutrient intake with the beautiful hues of nature!

Savor new flavors. Remember that it will take your taste buds time to adjust to eating plant-based foods after years of being bombarded with salt and sugar. At first things might taste bland, but with a little time, your preferences will change. You'll notice and appreciate and enjoy subtler flavors you might not have noticed before.

YOUR SPICE ARSENAL

Previously, your spice drawer was probably sparse or full of spices that were seldom used. Now it will be filled with spices that you will know intimately and use consistently. The meal plan uses the following spices across all four weeks. These will be listed in the "Staples to Check For" box in the weekly ingredients section.

- Black pepper
- Cayenne pepper
- Chili powder
- Curry powder
- Garlic powder
- Ground cinnamon
- Ground cumin
- Ground turmeric
- Italian seasoning
- Nutritional yeast
- Onion powder
- Red pepper flakes
- Smoked paprika

ABOUT THE RECIPES

With your success in mind, most recipes in this book, from the meal plans to the Bonus Recipes in chapter 8, have been designed to be as versatile and beginner-friendly as possible. Some will have extra-easy labels, like **5 Ingredients** (no more than five main ingredients, not counting salt, pepper, water, or cooking oil); **One Pot**, **One Pan**, or **One Bowl** (aside from a plate for batch cooking or a small bowl to mix ingredients, these only need one vessel to make); **Quick** (recipes take 30 minutes or less to prep and cook, from start to finish); and **No Cook** (no stovetop or oven required!). You'll also find tips and tricks along the way to help you get the most out of your cooking.

In addition, to help you pick dishes that fit your dietary needs, you'll find labels for recipes that are **gluten-free**, **nut-free**, **oil-free**, or **soy-free**. Although the US Food and Drug Administration labels coconuts as tree nuts, they are technically a seed or a tree fruit. Some folks with tree nut allergies may also react to coconuts; however, most can safely consume them since they lack many of the proteins present in tree nuts. If you have allergy concerns, please consult your doctor before adding any items to your diet. For gluten-free items, always make sure to check the ingredient packaging for a label to make sure they were processed in a gluten-free facility.

From cutting down prep time to simple ingredient swaps and flavor variations to information about ingredients you might not be familiar with and storage and reheating instructions, I've got you covered. Now let's get cooking!

Strawberry, Banana,
and Granola Yogurt
Bowls, page 32

CHAPTER FOUR

MEAL PLAN FOR DAYS 1 TO 7

ARE YOU READY TO DIVE HEADFIRST INTO PLANT-BASED EATING?
This first week's menu will ease you into the meal plan with some delicious and easy meals that will rev up your taste buds and excite you about the program.

29
Peanut Butter and Strawberry Jam Oatmeal

30
Tempeh "Bacon," Tomato, and Avocado Toasts

32
Strawberry, Banana, and Granola Yogurt Bowls

33
Smashed White Bean Salad Sammies

34
Brown Rice and Black Bean Veggie Burgers

36
Quick Creamy Herbed Tomato Soup

37
Hearty Black Bean and Corn Soup

38
Tofu and Zoodles Dinner Salad with Spicy Peanut Sauce

40
Roasted Root Vegetable Hash with Yogurt and Avocado

42
Butternut Squash and White Bean Mac and Cheeze

44
Creamy Curried Potatoes and Peas

46
Chickpea and Cauliflower Fajitas

47
Plant-Based Chocolate-Chunk Cookies

WEEK 1

	Breakfast	Lunch	Dinner
SUNDAY	Peanut Butter and Strawberry Jam Oatmeal (page 29)	Smashed White Bean Salad Sammies (page 33)	Brown Rice and Black Bean Veggie Burgers (page 34)
MONDAY	Strawberry, Banana, and Granola Yogurt Bowl (page 32)	Quick Creamy Herbed Tomato Soup (page 36)	Chickpea and Cauliflower Fajitas (page 46)
TUESDAY	Roasted Root Vegetable Hash with Yogurt and Avocado (page 40)	*Leftover* Chickpea and Cauliflower Fajitas	Butternut Squash and White Bean Mac and Cheeze (page 42)
WEDNESDAY	*Leftover* Peanut Butter and Strawberry Jam Oatmeal	*Leftover* Brown Rice and Black Bean Veggie Burgers	Creamy Curried Potatoes and Peas (page 44)
THURSDAY	*Leftover* Roasted Root Vegetable Hash with Yogurt and Sliced Avocado	*Leftover* Butternut Squash and White Bean Mac and Cheeze	Hearty Black Bean and Corn Soup (page 37)
FRIDAY	Tempeh "Bacon," Tomato, and Avocado Toasts (page 30)	*Leftover* Quick Creamy Herbed Tomato Soup with *Leftover* Tempeh "Bacon," Tomato, and Avocado Toasts	Tofu and Zoodles Dinner Salad with Spicy Peanut Sauce (page 38)
SATURDAY	Strawberry, Banana, and Granola Yogurt Bowls (page 32)	*Leftover* Hearty Black Bean and Corn Soup	*Leftover* Creamy Curried Potatoes and Peas

Weekly Dessert
Plant-Based Chocolate-Chunk Cookies (page 47)

Ingredients You'll Need

FRESH PRODUCE

Arugula (handful)

Avocados (3)

Banana (1)

Bell pepper, red (1)

Butternut squash (1)

Carrots, large (5)

Cauliflower (1 head)

Celery (3 stalks)

Cilantro (1 large bunch)

Cucumbers, Persian (2)

Garlic (8 cloves)

Ginger root (2 inches)

Lemon (1)

Limes (2)

Mint (1 small package)

Onions, yellow, small (4)

Potatoes, red, small (10; about 1¼ pounds)

Potatoes, yellow, medium (2)

Radishes (1 bunch)

Red cabbage, shredded (1 cup)

Salad greens, mixed (2 cups)

Scallion (1)

Strawberries (½ pint)

Sweet potatoes, medium (3)

Tomatoes, medium (2)

Zucchini, small (1)

Zucchini noodles (8 ounces)

CANNED, BOTTLED, AND JARRED

Black beans, 3 (15-ounce) cans

Cannellini beans, 2 (15-ounce) cans

Chickpeas, 1 (15-ounce) can

Maple syrup (1¼ cups)

Natural peanut butter (½ cup)

No-sugar-added strawberry jam (¼ cup)

Soy sauce, low-sodium, or gluten-free tamari (5 tablespoons)

Tahini (2 tablespoons)

Tomatoes, crushed, 2 (15-ounce) cans

Tomatoes, diced 1 (15-ounce) can

Tomato paste (3 tablespoons)

REFRIGERATED OR FROZEN

Brown rice, frozen (1½ cups)

Corn, frozen (1 cup)

Milk, plant-based, unsweetened (3½ cups)

Peas, frozen (1 cup)

Tempeh, 1 (8-ounce) package

Tofu, firm or extra-firm, 1 (16-ounce) package

Yogurt, plant-based, plain unsweetened (2¼ cups; about 18 ounces)

CONTINUED ▶

PANTRY

Avocado oil (2 tablespoons)

Baking soda (1 teaspoon)

Chocolate, vegan, refined-sugar free (½ cup), such as Lily's, Pasha, or Fine & Raw brands

Coconut oil (¼ cup)

Flaxseeds, ground (1 tablespoon)

Flour, whole-wheat (3 cups)

Granola (1 cup)

Nutritional yeast (2 tablespoons)

Pasta, whole-wheat shells (1 pound)

Rolled oats (2 cups)

Tapioca flour (1 tablespoon)

Vanilla extract (2 teaspoons)

OTHER

Bread, whole-grain (8 slices)

Burger buns, whole-wheat (4)

Tortillas, corn, 6 inches (12)

Staples to Check For: Black pepper, chili powder, ground cumin, curry powder, extra-virgin olive oil, garlic powder, Italian seasoning, olive oil cooking spray, onion powder, red pepper flakes, salt, smoked paprika

Prep This

- One batch of Strawberry Chia Jam (page 182) for the Peanut Butter and Strawberry Jam Oatmeal (page 29) for Sunday breakfast (optional)
- One batch Crispy, Crunchy Granola (page 184) for Strawberry, Banana, and Granola Yogurt Bowls (page 32) for Monday breakfast (optional)

PEANUT BUTTER AND STRAWBERRY JAM OATMEAL

5 INGREDIENTS, OIL-FREE, ONE POT, QUICK, SOY-FREE

COOK TIME: 20 minutes / **MAKES 4 SERVINGS**

Peanut butter and jelly are a match made in heaven. This sweet, slightly salty, and hearty breakfast will capture your heart and keep your belly full for hours. You can switch up your nut butters and your jam flavors to create nearly endless flavor possibilities.

2 cups rolled oats

4 cups water

½ cup unsweetened plant-based milk

1 tablespoon maple syrup

Pinch salt

4 tablespoons natural peanut butter, divided

4 tablespoons no-sugar-added strawberry jam or Strawberry Chia Jam (page 182), divided

1. In a medium saucepan, combine the oats and water and bring to a boil over medium-high heat. Lower the heat to medium-low and simmer, stirring often, until the oats are soft and creamy, about 15 minutes. Remove from the heat. Add the plant-based milk, maple syrup, and salt and stir well.

2. Divide the oatmeal among 4 bowls, top each with 1 tablespoon of peanut butter and 1 tablespoon of jam, and serve immediately.

3. The oatmeal can be stored in an airtight container in the refrigerator for up to 4 days. To serve, reheat the oatmeal in a medium saucepan over low heat with 2 tablespoons water to loosen it up, as oatmeal can get quite solid when chilled. Add the peanut butter and jam just before serving.

Cooking Tip: When buying peanut butter, be sure to check the ingredients. Look for varieties made with only peanuts and salt. Many brands add sugar and oil as fillers.

Per serving (1 cup): Calories: 284; Fat: 12g; Carbohydrates: 35g; Protein: 11g; Fiber: 6g; Sodium: 57mg

TEMPEH "BACON," TOMATO, AND AVOCADO TOASTS

NUT-FREE

PREP TIME: 5 minutes, plus 30 minutes to marinate
COOK TIME: 15 minutes / **MAKES 2 SERVINGS**

There are few meats that evoke such fervor as bacon. The good news is that the flavor can be mimicked in a plant-based way by marinating tempeh in sweet, smoky, and salty flavors. While the texture of tempeh is much different from the texture of pork, the essence is similar enough that when combined with creamy avocado and tomato, even a devout carnivore can be tempted to the plant side.

1 (8-ounce) package tempeh	1½ teaspoons smoked paprika
2 tablespoons avocado oil, divided	4 slices whole-grain bread
2 tablespoons maple syrup	1 medium tomato, thinly sliced
3 tablespoons low-sodium soy sauce or gluten-free tamari	1 avocado
	Salt
	Black pepper

1. Cut the tempeh through the middle to make 2 thinner pieces. Then cut each in half lengthwise and finally cut each piece in half horizontally. You should have 8 rectangles. I like to cut it this way rather than in long strips like bacon, because the tempeh can get crumbly if it is too long.

2. In a medium bowl, combine 1 tablespoon of avocado oil, the maple syrup, soy sauce, and smoked paprika and whisk until combined. Add the sliced tempeh to the bowl and gently mix until each slice is well coated. Cover with plastic wrap and refrigerate for at least 30 minutes.

3. Heat a 10-inch nonstick pan over medium heat. Pour in the remaining 1 tablespoon avocado oil. Arrange the tempeh slices in one layer in the pan and cook until each slice is brown and crispy, about 5 minutes per side. For even crispier "bacon," cook each side for an additional 5 minutes. Discard any leftover marinade.

4. While the tempeh cooks, toast 2 slices of the bread. Cut the avocado in half, and then quarter and peel the half without the pit. Tightly wrap the pitted half in plastic wrap and refrigerate for later use.

5. Top each slice of toast with 2 pieces of tempeh, 2 slices of tomato, and a quarter of the sliced avocado. Season with salt and black pepper to taste.

Ingredient Tip: Tempeh is a fermented soybean cake that is high in protein, fiber, and iron. It is firmer than tofu and has a stronger, nuttier taste. If the flavor is too strong for you, you can steam or boil it in water for 10 minutes before incorporating it into your recipes. This will mellow out its very distinctive flavor.

Leftovers Tip: This also works for a quick lunch that pairs perfectly with the Quick Creamy Herbed Tomato Soup (page 36). Refrigerate your leftover tempeh, tomato, and avocado separately. When it's lunchtime, microwave the tempeh until warmed through, and follow steps 4 and 5 as directed.

Per serving (1 toast): Calories: 396; Fat: 22g; Carbohydrates: 30g; Protein: 17g; Fiber: 6g; Sodium: 494mg

STRAWBERRY, BANANA, AND GRANOLA YOGURT BOWLS

5 INGREDIENTS, NO COOK, OIL-FREE, QUICK

PREP TIME: 10 minutes / **MAKES 2 SERVINGS**

When I first discovered the combo of yogurt, fresh fruit, and granola in college, I felt like I had hit the jackpot. I had finally found a breakfast that wasn't too sweet and could double as a good-for-you dessert. It's light enough not to weigh you down in the morning, but it's filling enough to fuel you until lunchtime. As a plant-based eater, I love eating variations of this nourishing and tasty bowl all week long.

2 cups plain plant-based yogurt

1 cup granola or Crispy, Crunchy Granola (page 184)

2 tablespoons maple syrup

1 cup sliced strawberries

1 medium banana, sliced

Divide the yogurt between 2 serving bowls. Top each bowl with ½ cup of granola and drizzle with 1 tablespoon of maple syrup. Divide the strawberries and bananas between the bowls and serve immediately.

Variation Tip: In winter when fresh fruit is not abundant, use 1 cup frozen blueberries or 2 tablespoons of your favorite jam instead of fresh fruit.

Per serving: Calories: 391; Fat: 8g; Carbohydrates: 66g; Protein: 12g; Fiber: 9g; Sodium: 195mg

SMASHED WHITE BEAN SALAD SAMMIES

NO COOK, NUT-FREE, OIL-FREE, QUICK, SOY-FREE

PREP TIME: 15 minutes / **MAKES 2 SANDWICHES**

This white bean salad is wonderfully fresh and simple. The flavors really complement one another, and when paired with arugula and sliced tomatoes, they make a Mediterranean-influenced masterpiece. You can enjoy it as a sandwich or mix everything up and eat it straight out of a bowl with some whole-grain crackers or over greens.

1 garlic clove, minced

2 tablespoons minced celery (about ½ stalk)

1 scallion, greens and white parts, minced

2 or 3 fresh mint leaves, finely chopped

1 (15-ounce) can cannellini beans, drained and rinsed

Juice of ½ large lemon

2 tablespoons tahini

Pinch ground cumin

Pinch salt, plus more as needed

Pinch red pepper flakes

4 slices whole-grain bread

1 handful arugula

1 medium tomato, sliced

1. In a large bowl, mix together the garlic, celery, scallion, and mint. Add the drained beans, lemon juice, tahini, cumin, salt, and red pepper flakes and stir, mashing the beans with a fork, until combined. The mixture will be rustic and chunky.

2. To make each sandwich, spread about ½ cup of filling onto 1 slice of bread, top with arugula and tomato slices, sprinkle with a little salt (if desired), and top with another piece of bread. Refrigerate leftover filling for up to 4 days.

Variation Tip: Try a can of chickpeas instead of cannellini beans. Or add 6 to 8 pitted and chopped kalamata olives for an extra tang.

Per serving (1 sandwich): Calories: 397; Fat: 12g; Carbohydrates: 57g; Protein: 20g; Fiber: 7g; Sodium: 575mg

BROWN RICE AND BLACK BEAN VEGGIE BURGERS

NUT-FREE, SOY-FREE

PREP TIME: 15 minutes / **COOK TIME:** 20 minutes / **MAKES 6 PATTIES**

Although there are many options for prepared frozen plant-based burgers, it's invaluable to have a good homemade recipe in your repertoire. These get a meaty taste from the smoked paprika and brown rice and will crisp slightly around the edges. Serve them on a bun topped with your favorite fixings, like Plant-Based Mayo (page 178), sliced tomato, and onion, or on top of a fresh green salad with a drizzle of Lemon Aioli (page 142).

1 cup water

1 sweet potato, peeled and cut into ½-inch pieces (about 1 cup)

Olive oil cooking spray

1 (15-ounce) can black beans, drained and rinsed

1½ cups frozen brown rice

1 tablespoon garlic powder

1 tablespoon onion powder

½ teaspoon smoked paprika

1 teaspoon tapioca flour

1 teaspoon ground flaxseeds

1 tablespoon nutritional yeast

¼ teaspoon salt

4 whole-wheat burger buns, for serving

1. In a medium saucepan, bring the water to a boil over high heat. Add the sweet potato and cook until it's easily pierced with a fork, about 10 minutes. Drain and set aside to cool.

2. Preheat the oven to 425°F. Spray a sheet pan with olive oil cooking spray.

3. In a large bowl, combine the sweet potato and black beans and, using a fork or potato masher, mash until they are well combined but still chunky. Add the frozen rice, garlic powder, onion powder, smoked paprika, tapioca flour, ground flaxseeds, nutritional yeast, and salt and mix until well combined. The mixture will be very sticky.

4. Using your hands, form the mixture into 6 equal patties. Put the patties onto the prepared sheet pan and bake for 10 minutes. Flip the burgers and continue to bake for another 10 minutes, until browned and crispy. Arrange on buns and serve.

Leftovers Tip: Let the patties cool completely, wrap them individually in plastic wrap, and refrigerate for up to 5 days or freeze for up to 3 months. To reheat, thaw in the refrigerator and pan-fry or microwave until warmed through.

Per serving (1 patty): Calories: 142; Fat: 1g; Carbohydrates: 28g; Protein: 6g; Fiber: 6g; Sodium: 112mg

QUICK CREAMY HERBED TOMATO SOUP

GLUTEN-FREE, NUT-FREE, QUICK

PREP TIME: 5 minutes / **COOK TIME:** 15 minutes / **MAKES 4 SERVINGS**

This dish is a plant-based version of a customer favorite that was on my menu for many years. The addition of herbs and pan-roasted garlic gives this staple a fresh take and depth of flavor—and as an added bonus, your kitchen will smell incredible as it's cooking! For a heartier meal, pair the soup with Smashed White Bean Salad Sammies (page 33).

2 teaspoons extra-virgin olive oil

4 garlic cloves, roughly chopped

2 (15-ounce) cans crushed
  tomatoes

½ teaspoon maple syrup

2 cups plain unsweetened
  plant-based milk

1 teaspoon Italian seasoning

2 tablespoons roughly chopped
  fresh mint

½ teaspoon salt

Black pepper

1. In a medium saucepan, heat the oil over medium heat. Add the garlic and cook it until it is fragrant and beginning to turn golden, about 2 minutes. Remove from the heat and let cool.

2. In a blender or food processor, combine the tomatoes, maple syrup, plant-based milk, Italian seasoning, mint, salt, and cooled garlic and blend until smooth.

3. Return the mixture to the saucepan and bring to a boil over high heat. Lower the heat to medium-low and simmer, stirring occasionally, for 5 minutes. Ladle into bowls, sprinkle with black pepper, and serve.

Leftovers Tip: Store leftovers in an airtight container in the refrigerator for up to 5 days. To reheat, transfer to a saucepan and heat over medium heat until hot.

Variation Tip: Any fresh herbs will taste great in this recipe. I like to use whichever ones I have on hand to avoid food waste. My favorites are basil, oregano, and cilantro.

Per serving: Calories: 126; Fat: 5g; Carbohydrates: 17g; Protein: 6g; Fiber: 5g; Sodium: 598mg

HEARTY BLACK BEAN AND CORN SOUP

GLUTEN-FREE, NUT-FREE, ONE POT, SOY-FREE

PREP TIME: 10 minutes / **COOK TIME:** 30 minutes / **MAKES 4 SERVINGS**

Since I'm originally from Massachusetts, where the winters are blustery cold, I have a deep appreciation for a bowl of hot soup. This soup is super hearty and packed full of vegetables. The flavor profile is Southwestern with zippy cilantro and smoky tomato undertones.

2 tablespoons extra-virgin olive oil

1 small yellow onion, diced small

2 large carrots, peeled and cut into thin rounds

2 celery stalks, diced small

1 (15-ounce) can diced tomatoes, or 2 medium tomatoes, cut into ½-inch pieces

2 small red potatoes, cut into small cubes

2 (15-ounce) cans black beans, drained and rinsed

1 cup frozen corn

8 cups water

1 teaspoon smoked paprika

1 teaspoon salt

1 teaspoon garlic powder

1 small zucchini, cut into small cubes

1 tablespoon finely chopped fresh cilantro

1. In a large saucepan, heat the oil over medium heat. Add the onion, carrots, and celery and cook until the onions are fragrant and the vegetables are starting to get tender, 5 to 7 minutes.

2. Add the tomatoes and cook, stirring occasionally, for 5 minutes. Add the potatoes, beans, corn, and water and stir until combined. Raise the heat to high, bring to a rolling boil, and cook for 5 minutes.

3. Add the smoked paprika, salt, garlic powder, zucchini, and cilantro and stir until combined. Lower the heat to medium-low and simmer the soup until the vegetables are fork-tender, about 15 minutes. Serve hot.

Per serving: Calories: 380; Fat: 8g; Carbohydrates: 63g; Protein: 16g; Fiber: 16g; Sodium: 639mg

TOFU AND ZOODLES DINNER SALAD WITH SPICY PEANUT SAUCE

GLUTEN-FREE, QUICK

PREP TIME: 10 minutes / **COOK TIME:** 20 minutes / **MAKES 2 SERVINGS**

I admit, when I first heard about zucchini noodles I doubted how good they could be, but since I never met a veggie that I don't like, I gave them a try. I was pleasantly surprised by the flavor, and after many experiments I realized that raw "zoodles" were the closest option to replicate a regular noodle texture. In this recipe, I pair them with baked tofu; a sweet, spicy, and salty peanut sauce; crunchy cabbage and carrots; and the freshness of mint and cilantro. It's a salad fit to be called an entrée.

FOR THE TOFU

Olive oil cooking spray

1 (16-ounce package) firm or extra-firm tofu

Salt

FOR THE PEANUT SAUCE

3 tablespoons natural peanut butter

2 tablespoons low-sodium soy sauce or gluten-free tamari

2 teaspoons maple syrup

Juice of 2 limes

Pinch red pepper flakes (optional)

FOR THE ZOODLE SALAD

2 small Persian cucumbers, thinly sliced

1 large carrot, peeled and julienned

5 fresh mint leaves, julienned

1 handful fresh cilantro, chopped

6 to 8 ounces store-bought zucchini noodles (about 2 small zucchini)

2 cups mixed salad greens

1 cup shredded red cabbage

1. **Prepare the tofu:** Preheat the oven to 425°F. Spray a sheet pan with olive oil cooking spray.

2. Drain the tofu and place it on a plate lined with a clean kitchen towel. Place another plate on top of the tofu to press out a bit more of the liquid. Pat the tofu dry with a clean kitchen towel. Cut the tofu into small cubes.

3. Spread out the tofu in a single layer on the sheet pan, sprinkle with salt, and bake for 10 minutes. Using a spatula, flip the tofu and continue to bake for another 10 minutes.

4. **Make the peanut sauce:** In a medium bowl, whisk together the peanut butter, soy sauce, maple syrup, lime juice, and red pepper flakes (if using). Add water, 1 tablespoon at a time, and whisk until the sauce is thick but still pourable. Set aside.

5. **Make the salad:** Put the cucumbers, carrot, mint, and cilantro in a large bowl. Add the zucchini noodles, greens, and cabbage and toss until combined.

6. To serve, portion the salad into bowls. Divide the tofu equally among the bowls and top with the peanut sauce.

Leftovers Tip: Store ingredients in separate airtight containers. Once dressed, the vegetables will begin to break down. Undressed, the ingredients will last for up to 3 days in the refrigerator.

Variation Tip: Substitute ½ pound of your favorite noodles for the zucchini noodles. Cook the noodles according to the package instructions, rinse with cold water, and toss with 1 tablespoon of olive oil to prevent sticking.

Per serving: Calories: 465; Fat: 26g; Carbohydrates: 34g; Protein: 35g; Fiber: 7g; Sodium: 583mg

ROASTED ROOT VEGETABLE HASH WITH YOGURT AND AVOCADO

GLUTEN-FREE, NUT-FREE, ONE PAN

PREP TIME: 15 minutes / **COOK TIME:** 30 minutes / **MAKES 4 SERVINGS**

Hearty breakfast hashes are a classic morning favorite. My plant-based version maximizes your vegetable consumption by including ample root veggies and squash in addition to potatoes. Rather than cooking on a griddle or stovetop, which can require lots of oil, I opt for the mighty sheet pan. Substitute any vegetable for the same amount of hard squash, like kabocha and delicata or root vegetables like beets, parsnips, and turnips. Just remember the golden rule of sheet-pan cooking: cut quick-cooking veggies larger and ones that take longer smaller so everything finishes cooking at the same time.

2 teaspoons extra-virgin olive oil

1 small yellow onion, cut into ½-inch pieces

½ medium butternut squash (about 1 pound), peeled, seeded, and cut into 1½-inch cubes

2 large carrots, peeled and cut into 1-inch rounds

2 medium sweet potatoes (about ½ pound), cut into 1½-inch cubes

2 medium yellow potatoes (about ½ pound), cut into 1½-inch cubes

1 bunch small red or pink radishes, trimmed and halved

1 teaspoon garlic powder

1 teaspoon smoked paprika

1 teaspoon salt

4 tablespoons plain plant-based yogurt, for serving

1 avocado, peeled, pitted, quartered, and thinly sliced, for serving

Black pepper

1. Preheat the oven to 400°F. Grease a sheet pan with the olive oil, making sure to spread it into the edges.

2. Combine the onion, butternut squash, carrots, sweet potatoes, yellow potatoes, and radishes on the sheet pan and sprinkle with garlic powder, smoked paprika, and salt. Using your hands, toss the vegetables until evenly coated with the oil and spices.

3. Bake for 20 minutes. Using a spatula, flip the vegetables and bake for another 10 minutes, or until the vegetables can be easily pierced with a fork.

4. Divide the hash among plates and top each portion with 1 tablespoon of yogurt, a quarter of the avocado slices, and black pepper to taste.

Leftovers Tip: Store the hash separate from the yogurt and avocado slices. Since the toppings are chilled, you don't want to warm them. Reheat the hash in the microwave on high for 2 minutes or in the oven at 400°F for 10 minutes.

Per serving: Calories: 325; Fat: 10g; Carbohydrates: 56g; Protein: 7g; Fiber: 12g; Sodium: 660mg

BUTTERNUT SQUASH AND WHITE BEAN MAC AND CHEEZE

NUT-FREE, OIL-FREE, QUICK

PREP TIME: 10 minutes / **COOK TIME:** 20 minutes / **MAKES 4 SERVINGS**

The traditional mac and cheese is filling, affordable, and quick to make—and this plant-based version checks all those boxes, too. The combo of creamy white beans, sweet butternut squash, and "cheesy" nutritional yeast makes this a fake that won't leave you longing for the old-school powdered stuff. To cut down the prep time even more, opt for precut squash. If using frozen squash, make sure to cook for half the time given below.

1 pound whole-wheat pasta shells

½ cup plus 2 teaspoons water, divided

½ medium butternut squash, peeled, seeded, and cut into 1-inch cubes (about 2 cups)

1 (15-ounce) can cannellini beans, drained and rinsed

1 cup unsweetened plant-based milk

1 teaspoon salt

½ teaspoon onion powder

½ teaspoon garlic powder

1 tablespoon nutritional yeast

2 teaspoons tapioca flour

Pinch red pepper flakes (optional)

1. Bring a large pot of water to a boil over high heat. Pour in the pasta and cook according to the package instructions. Drain the pasta and return it to the pot.

2. In a medium saucepan, bring ½ cup of water to a boil over high heat. Add the butternut squash and cook until the squash is fork-tender, about 8 minutes. Do not drain.

3. In a blender or food processor, combine the squash and its cooking water, beans, and milk and blend until smooth. Add the salt, onion powder, garlic powder, and nutritional yeast and blend again.

4. Pour the sauce back into the saucepan and bring it to a boil over medium-high heat, stirring often. This will happen in 3 to 5 minutes.

5. In a small bowl, combine the tapioca flour and the remaining 2 teaspoons water to make a slurry. Add the slurry to the bubbling sauce and cook, stirring constantly, until the sauce thickens, about 3 minutes. Remove from the heat.

6. Add the sauce to the pot with the pasta and stir well until evenly coated. Serve with a pinch of crushed red pepper on top (if using).

Leftovers Tip: Refrigerate for up to 3 days. Microwave with 2 tablespoons of water in 2-minute increments, stirring in between, until heated through, or cook in a skillet over low heat for 5 minutes, stirring often.

Variation Tip: Add some broccoli or cauliflower florets to the pasta during the last couple minutes of cooking. Drain with the pasta and combine with the sauce as instructed. This dish tastes great with a scoop of Black and White Bean Chili (page 90) or Crispy Baked Chickpeas (page 146).

Per serving (2 cups): Calories: 553; Fat: 3g; Carbohydrates: 114g; Protein: 25g; Fiber: 17g; Sodium: 625mg

CREAMY CURRIED POTATOES AND PEAS

GLUTEN-FREE, NUT-FREE, ONE PAN, SOY-FREE

PREP TIME: 15 minutes / **COOK TIME:** 30 minutes / **MAKES 4 SERVINGS**

Growing up, I had zero exposure to the delicious flavors of India. After my first taste of curry, I was enamored. These days curries are a staple in my diet and some of the most-loved recipes on my blog, *Better Food Guru*. Here, potatoes are bathed in a creamy, spicy gravy, and the peas add a component of sweetness that is the perfect complement to the heat. For some added bulk, try it over brown rice or quinoa.

1 tablespoon extra-virgin olive oil

8 small red potatoes (about 1 pound), diced small

3 garlic cloves, minced

1 (2-inch) piece fresh ginger, peeled and minced

1 small yellow onion, cut into ¼-inch pieces

3 teaspoons curry powder

2 cups water

1 cup frozen peas

3 tablespoons tomato paste

1 teaspoon salt, plus more as needed

Black pepper

Red pepper flakes (optional)

¼ cup chopped fresh cilantro, for garnish

1. In a large saucepan or wok, heat the oil over medium heat. Add the potatoes and cook, stirring often, until they start to brown, about 10 minutes. Push the potatoes to one side of the pan, then add the garlic, ginger, and onion and cook, stirring occasionally, until very fragrant, about 5 minutes. Stir the onion mixture with the potatoes until combined.

2. Add the curry powder and water and stir until combined. Raise the heat to high and bring to a boil. Lower the heat to medium and cook, stirring occasionally, until the potatoes are fork-tender, 10 to 15 minutes.

3. Stir in the peas, tomato paste, and salt and cook, stirring occasionally, until the liquid reduces to a creamy sauce, 4 to 5 minutes.

4. Taste and season with salt and black pepper. Sprinkle with red pepper flakes (if using) and the cilantro.

Variation Tip: Add 2 cups of chopped fresh spinach during the last few minutes of cooking or stir in 1 (15-ounce) can drained chickpeas during step 2. If you're a fan of spicy food, add ½ teaspoon cayenne pepper in step 2.

Per serving: Calories: 323; Fat: 4g; Carbohydrates: 65g; Protein: 9g; Fiber: 9g; Sodium: 654mg

CHICKPEA AND CAULIFLOWER FAJITAS

GLUTEN-FREE, NUT-FREE, ONE PAN, QUICK, SOY-FREE

PREP TIME: 10 minutes / **COOK TIME:** 30 minutes / **MAKES 4 SERVINGS**

I tried my first fajita platter back when I was a teenager living in rural Massachusetts and was immediately smitten. This plant-based version with chickpeas and cauliflower is quick to make and eclipses traditional fajitas in both flavor and nutrition.

1 tablespoon extra-virgin olive oil

½ large head cauliflower, cut into small florets (about 2 cups)

1 small yellow onion, thinly sliced

1 red bell pepper, seeded and thinly sliced

1 (15-ounce) can chickpeas, drained and rinsed

1 teaspoon chili powder

½ teaspoon smoked paprika

½ teaspoon garlic powder

1 teaspoon salt

12 (6-inch) soft corn tortillas, for serving

1 avocado, pitted, peeled, quartered, and thinly sliced, or Super-Simple Guacamole (page 171), for serving

½ bunch cilantro, chopped, for serving

1. In a large sauté pan, heat the oil over medium heat. Add the cauliflower and cook until it begins to brown, about 5 minutes. Add the onion and cook, stirring occasionally, for 5 minutes. Add the bell pepper and cook, stirring occasionally, until the cauliflower is fork-tender, about 5 minutes.

2. Add the chickpeas, chili powder, smoked paprika, garlic powder, and salt and stir until combined. Cook until the spices flavor the mixture, about 5 minutes. Transfer the fajita mixture to a serving bowl.

3. Wipe out the sauté pan with a paper towel and warm the tortillas over medium heat until they are pliable, about 2 minutes per side.

4. Divide the filling among the tortillas, top each one with 2 or 3 slices of avocado and some chopped cilantro, and serve.

Per serving (3 fajitas): Calories: 500; Fat: 18g; Carbohydrates: 73g; Protein: 15g; Fiber: 13g; Sodium: 1,023mg

PLANT-BASED CHOCOLATE-CHUNK COOKIES

NUT-FREE, QUICK, SOY-FREE

PREP TIME: 10 minutes / **COOK TIME:** 15 minutes / **MAKES 18 COOKIES**

This plant-based cookie showcases the traditional flavors without all the butter and refined sugar. Gluten-free baking flours work great here and make these treats even more allergen friendly.

2 teaspoons ground flaxseeds

2 tablespoons cold water

¼ cup coconut oil

3 cups whole-wheat flour

1 teaspoon baking soda

½ teaspoon salt

¼ cup extra-virgin olive oil

¾ cup maple syrup

2 teaspoons vanilla extract

5 teaspoons water

½ cup vegan refined-sugar-free chocolate-chunks

1. Preheat the oven to 350°F. Line a sheet pan with parchment paper.

2. In a medium bowl, combine the ground flaxseeds and cold water to make 2 "flax eggs." Let the mixture sit for 5 minutes.

3. In a small microwave-safe bowl, microwave the coconut oil for 25 to 30 seconds, until it becomes a liquid. Set aside.

4. In a large bowl, mix together the flour, baking soda, and salt. Add the melted coconut oil, olive oil, maple syrup, and vanilla to the flax eggs and mix until well combined.

5. Add the wet ingredients to the flour mixture and mix until well combined. The batter will be a little dry, so add the water and mix well. Fold in the chocolate chips.

6. Roll the dough into 2-inch balls and put them on the prepared sheet pan. Flatten them slightly with your fingers. Bake for 15 minutes. Let cool completely, and store at room temperature for up to 1 week.

Per serving (2 cookies): Calories: 369; Fat: 18g; Carbohydrates: 49g; Protein: 7g; Fiber: 6g; Sodium: 275mg

Roasted Cauliflower
Bowls with Spicy
Garlic-Tahini Sauce,
page 70

MEAL PLAN FOR DAYS 8 TO 14

WEEK 2

	Breakfast	Lunch	Dinner
SUNDAY	Sweet Potato Toasts with Avocado Mash and Tahini (page 56)	Loaded Chickpea Noodle Soup (page 60)	Fettuccine with Creamy Cashew Alfredo (page 66)
MONDAY	*Leftover* Sweet Potato Toasts with Avocado Mash and Tahini	*Leftover* Fettuccine with Creamy Cashew Alfredo	Tempeh and Lentil Sloppy Joes (page 65)
TUESDAY	Spiced Tofu and Potato Breakfast Burritos (page 58)	*Leftover* Loaded Chickpea Noodle Soup	Vegetable Korma Curry (page 68)
WEDNESDAY	Zucchini Bread Oatmeal (page 54)	Chickpea Curry Salad Sandwiches (page 64)	Spicy Butternut Squash Bisque (page 62)
THURSDAY	*Leftover* Zucchini Bread Oatmeal	*Leftover* Tempeh and Lentil Sloppy Joes	Roasted Cauliflower Bowls with Spicy Garlic-Tahini Sauce (page 70)
FRIDAY	Blueberry and Peanut Butter Parfait Bowls (page 55)	*Leftover* Chickpea Curry Salad Sandwiches	Tempeh and Walnut "Chorizo" Tacos (page 72)
SATURDAY	*Leftover* Spiced Tofu and Potato Breakfast Burritos	*Leftover* Spicy Butternut Squash Bisque	*Leftover* Vegetable Korma Curry

Weekly Dessert
Chocolate Tahini Muffins (page 74)

Ingredients You'll Need

FRESH PRODUCE

Apple (1)

Arugula (4 cups; 3 to 4 ounces)

Avocados (3)

Bananas (2)

Bell pepper, red (1)

Blueberries (½ cup)

Broccoli, florets, fresh or frozen (2 cups)

Butternut squash (1)

Carrots, large (3)

Cauliflower (1 head)

Celery (2 stalks)

Cilantro (1 large bunch)

Cucumber, Persian (1)

Garlic (16 cloves; about 2 heads)

Ginger (2 to 3 inches; 2 tablespoons chopped)

Jalapeño pepper (1)

Lemons (2)

Lettuce, iceberg (1 head)

Onion, yellow, small (3)

Potatoes, medium (3)

Spinach, baby (4 cups)

Sweet potatoes, medium (6)

Tomatoes, medium (7)

Zucchini, medium (1)

CANNED, BOTTLED, AND JARRED

Cannellini beans, 1 (15-ounce) can

Chickpeas, 2 (15-ounce) cans

Coconut milk, light unsweetened, 1 (15-ounce) can

Peanut butter, natural (2 tablespoons)

Tomato paste (5 tablespoons; about 1 small can)

REFRIGERATED OR FROZEN

Green beans, frozen (½ cup)

Mayonnaise, plant-based (2 teaspoons)

Milk, plant-based, unsweetened (6 cups; 48 ounces)

Peas, frozen (1 cup)

Salsa (1¼ cups)

Sriracha (1 teaspoon)

Tahini (½ cup)

Tempeh, 2 (8-ounce) packages

Tofu, extra-firm, 1 (16-ounce) package

Yogurt, plant-based, plain unsweetened (2½ cups; about 20 ounces)

CONTINUED ▶

PANTRY

Apple cider vinegar
(1 tablespoon)

Brown rice
(3 cups cooked)

Cashews, raw (2 cups)

Cocoa powder,
unsweetened (¼ cup)

Flaxseeds, ground
(2 tablespoons)

Flour, whole-wheat
(2½ cups)

Granola (1 cup)

Hemp hearts
(3 tablespoons)

Ketchup, sugar-free
(3 tablespoons)

Lentils, dried (¾ cup)

Molasses (1 tablespoon)

Maple syrup (about
¾ cup)

Nutritional yeast (about
½ cup)

Oats, rolled (2 cups)

Olives, kalamata (10)

Pasta, elbows or rotini,
whole-grain (1 pound)

Pasta, fettuccine,
whole-grain (1 pound)

Pepitas (1/4 cup)

Raisins (1 cup)

Sesame seeds
(2 tablespoons)

Tapioca flour
(1 teaspoon)

Walnuts (1½ cups; about
6 ounces)

OTHER

Bread, whole-wheat
(4 slices)

Burger buns,
whole-wheat (4)

Red miso paste
(4 teaspoons)

Tortillas, corn,
6 inches (8)

Tortillas, whole-wheat
flour, 12 inches (4)

Staples to Check For: Baking powder, black pepper, cayenne pepper, chili powder, coconut oil, ground cumin, curry powder, extra-virgin olive oil, garlic powder, ground turmeric, Italian seasoning, olive oil cooking spray, onion powder, red pepper flakes, salt, smoked paprika

Prep This

- One batch Nutty Plant-Based Parmesan (page 174) for Fettuccine with Creamy Cashew Alfredo (page 66) for Sunday's dinner (optional)

- Monday: Prepare 3 cups of cooked brown rice for serving with the Vegetable Korma Curry (page 68) and Roasted Cauliflower Bowls with Spicy Garlic-Tahini Sauce (page 70).

- Monday: One batch Pico de Gallo (page 172) for Spiced Tofu and Potato Breakfast Burritos (page 58). Refrigerate leftovers in a covered container and use for Tempeh and Walnut "Chorizo" Tacos (page 72) (optional).

- One batch Plant-Based Mayo (page 178) for Chickpea Curry Salad (page 64) for Wednesday's and Friday's lunches (optional)

- One batch Crispy Baked Chickpeas (page 146) for Spicy Butternut Squash Bisque (page 62) for Wednesday's dinner and Friday's lunch (optional)

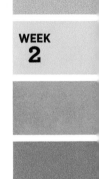

WEEK
2

ZUCCHINI BREAD OATMEAL

PREP TIME: 5 minutes / **COOK TIME:** 20 minutes / **MAKES 4 SERVINGS**

Since many people struggle with getting the recommended five servings of fruit and vegetables per day, I often find ways to add hidden veggies into my recipes and meals. The idea of adding zucchini to your oatmeal might sound strange, but much like zucchini bread, you'll hardly notice it in the finished product. Not only will adding zucchini up the fiber content of your breakfast, but it is also full of antioxidants, so it's a great way to start the day.

2 cups rolled oats

1 medium zucchini, grated

4 cups water

½ cup unsweetened
    plant-based milk

1 tablespoon ground cinnamon

½ cup raisins

1 tablespoon maple syrup

Pinch salt

2 medium bananas, sliced

4 tablespoons chopped walnuts
    (optional)

1. In a medium saucepan over medium-high, combine the oats, zucchini, and water and bring to a boil. Lower the heat to medium-low and simmer, stirring often, until the oats are soft and creamy, about 15 minutes. Remove from the heat, add the plant-based milk, cinnamon, raisins, maple syrup, and salt and stir well.

2. Divide the oatmeal among 4 bowls and top each portion with ½ sliced banana and 1 tablespoon of walnuts (if using).

Leftovers Tip: Refrigerate the oatmeal, without the bananas and walnuts, for up to 3 days. To reheat, warm the oatmeal on the stovetop until heated through and top with the bananas and walnuts.

Per serving (1 cup): Calories: 301; Fat: 4g; Carbohydrates: 62g; Protein: 9g; Fiber: 8g; Sodium: 62mg

BLUEBERRY AND PEANUT BUTTER PARFAIT BOWLS

NO COOK, OIL-FREE, QUICK

PREP TIME: 10 minutes / **MAKES 2 SERVINGS**

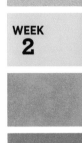

This is an ultra-quick and filling breakfast that will keep you fueled for hours. The combo of savory nut butter with the creamy yogurt and crunchy granola is über-satisfying. The addition of sweet fresh blueberries, mild and crunchy walnuts, and a drizzle of maple syrup packs a mega dose of morning antioxidants that will set you up for a day of sweet success. For a more impressive presentation, you can layer each ingredient in a glass or jar—this also is a great way to take it to work for a healthy breakfast on the go.

2 cups plain plant-based yogurt

1 cup store-bought granola or Crispy, Crunchy Granola (page 184)

2 tablespoons maple syrup

½ cup fresh blueberries

2 tablespoons roughly chopped walnuts

2 tablespoons natural peanut butter

1. Divide the yogurt between 2 bowls. Top each with half the granola and drizzle with 1 tablespoon maple syrup.

2. Top each bowl with half the blueberries, 1 tablespoon of walnuts, and 1 tablespoon peanut butter.

Variation Tip: This is an easily customizable and versatile breakfast treat. Switch out the blueberries and use whatever sweet and juicy fruits are in season. Stone fruits like peaches, nectarines, and apricots work very well, or try cherries, strawberries, and raspberries.

Per serving (1 cup): Calories: 567; Fat: 24g; Carbohydrates: 75g; Protein: 17g; Fiber: 13g; Sodium: 115mg

SWEET POTATO TOASTS WITH AVOCADO MASH AND TAHINI

GLUTEN-FREE, NUT-FREE, SOY-FREE

PREP TIME: 10 minutes / **COOK TIME:** 30 minutes / **MAKES 4 SERVINGS**

I discovered sweet potato toasts a few years ago when I was cutting down on my gluten intake. They make a tasty vehicle for a layered veggie toast that is delightfully different from the standard base. These versatile and filling toasts are also delicious with a sweet combo of nut butter and sliced apples, pears, or fresh peaches. For another savory option, try hummus topped with sautéed mushrooms.

FOR THE SWEET POTATO TOASTS

Olive oil cooking spray

4 medium sweet potatoes

Salt

FOR THE AVOCADO MASH

2 medium avocados, pitted and peeled

Juice of ½ lemon

Pinch salt

FOR SERVING

2 ounces arugula (about 2 cups)

8 teaspoons tahini

8 teaspoons hemp hearts

Pinch red pepper flakes (optional)

1. **Make the sweet potato toasts:** Preheat the oven to 400°F. Spray a sheet pan with olive oil cooking spray.

2. Cut the sweet potatoes lengthwise into ½-inch-thick slices (4 per potato).

3. Arrange the sweet potato slices in a single layer on the prepared sheet pan and sprinkle with salt. Bake for 15 minutes. Turn the slices over and continue to bake for another 15 minutes, or until the potatoes are slightly browned and crispy on the outside and soft in the middle.

4. **Make the avocado mash:** In a bowl, mash the avocados with a fork. Add the lemon juice and salt and stir until combined.

5. **Assemble the toasts:** Spread 1 teaspoon of avocado mash over each sweet potato toast. For each, add about 5 arugula leaves, drizzle with ½ teaspoon of tahini, and top with ½ teaspoon of hemp hearts. Add a pinch of red pepper flakes (if using).

Leftovers Tip: Wrap the sweet potato toasts tightly with plastic wrap and refrigerate for up to 5 days. Store the avocado mash in an airtight container and place plastic wrap directly on the mash before covering to avoid the browning. Microwave the toasts for 90 seconds before topping.

Per serving (4 toasts): Calories: 375; Fat: 23g; Carbohydrates: 38g; Protein: 7g; Fiber: 12g; Sodium: 113mg

SPICED TOFU AND POTATO BREAKFAST BURRITOS

NUT-FREE

PREP TIME: 10 minutes / **COOK TIME:** 25 minutes / **MAKES 4 BURRITOS**

In my opinion, the breakfast burrito may be one of the best culinary discoveries of the last century. Not only is it an amazingly convenient and portable meal, but it's also one of the most delicious ways to start your day. In this burrito, eggs are replaced with tofu, which is scrambled with spices, tomatoes, and potatoes, then slathered in salsa.

1 tablespoon extra-virgin olive oil

1 (16-ounce) package extra-firm tofu, drained and crumbled

2 medium potatoes, diced small

½ teaspoon salt

½ teaspoon garlic powder

½ teaspoon smoked paprika

½ teaspoon ground turmeric

2 medium tomatoes, chopped small

1 cup water

4 cups roughly chopped baby spinach

4 (12-inch) whole-wheat flour tortillas, for serving

1 avocado, peeled, pitted, and quartered, divided, for serving

4 tablespoons store-bought salsa or Pico de Gallo (page 172), for serving

1. In a medium saucepan, heat the oil over medium heat. Add the tofu and cook until it browns a little, about 5 minutes.

2. Add the potatoes and cook, stirring often, for about 5 minutes. Add the salt, garlic powder, smoked paprika, and turmeric and stir until the tofu and potatoes are well coated. Add the tomatoes and cook until they release their juices and the potatoes begin to soften, about 5 minutes.

3. Add the water and bring the mixture to a boil. Cook until the potatoes are fork-tender, 5 to 8 minutes. The liquid will reduce, though the scramble should be saucy, not too dry. Turn off the heat, add the baby spinach, and stir until it wilts.

4. Put the tortillas on a microwave-safe plate and microwave, uncovered, for about 30 seconds, until they are softened.

5. To assemble the burritos, place a quarter of the scramble in the center of each tortilla. Top with a quarter of the avocado and 1 tablespoon of salsa. Fold in the sides of the tortilla, and then roll it up from the bottom, wrapping it tightly around the filling.

Leftovers Tip: Cut the avocado in half, leaving the pit intact. Cover the exposed flesh with a little olive oil, wrap it tightly in plastic wrap, and refrigerate. Store all burrito components separately to avoid soggy tortillas.

Variation Tip: Add mushrooms or cauliflower, or instead of potatoes, use 1 (15-ounce) can black beans or pinto beans, drained and rinsed. Toss in some leftover quinoa or rice and forgo the tortillas to make a hearty burrito bowl.

Per serving (1 burrito): Calories: 576; Fat: 26g; Carbohydrates: 68g; Protein: 24g; Fiber: 16g; Sodium: 884mg

LOADED CHICKPEA NOODLE SOUP

NUT-FREE

PREP TIME: 10 minutes / **COOK TIME:** 30 minutes / **MAKES 4 SERVINGS**

Most of us grew up eating chicken noodle soup in the winter or anytime we had a cold. This soup evokes that same comfort-in-a-bowl feeling but with all plant-based ingredients. Red miso paste gives the broth a deep, complex flavor, and the addition of potatoes, chickpeas, and sweet potatoes results in a hearty and robust bowl of soup that is both delicious and nutritious.

1 pound whole-grain elbow or rotini pasta

1 tablespoon extra-virgin olive oil

2 garlic cloves, minced

½ small yellow onion, chopped

3 large carrots, peeled and cut into thin rounds

1 celery stalk, cut into small pieces

1 medium potato, peeled and diced

1 medium sweet potato, peeled and diced

2 medium tomatoes, chopped

1 (15-ounce) can chickpeas, drained and rinsed

1 tablespoon Italian seasoning

1 teaspoon salt

4 cups water

1 tablespoon red miso paste

¼ teaspoon black pepper

1. Bring a large pot of water to a boil over high heat. Add the pasta and cook according to the package instructions. Drain and set aside.

2. In a large saucepan, heat the olive oil over medium heat. Add the garlic and onion and cook until fragrant, about 5 minutes. Add the carrots and celery and cook until the vegetables begin to soften, about 5 minutes.

3. Add the potato, sweet potato, and tomatoes, lower the heat to low, and cook, stirring often, until the tomatoes release their juices, about 5 minutes.

4. Add the chickpeas, Italian seasoning, salt, and water and bring to a boil over high heat. Lower the heat to medium-low and simmer until the vegetables are fork-tender, about 10 minutes. Remove from the heat. Add the miso and pepper and stir until the miso dissolves. To serve, top each portion with a quarter of the noodles.

Cooking Tip: Make the soup in an Instant Pot: Press sauté, add the garlic, onion, and olive oil, and cook about 2 minutes. Add the carrots, celery, potato, sweet potato, and tomatoes and sauté for about 5 minutes. Add the water, chickpeas, Italian seasoning, and salt and stir until combined. Seal the lid and set the Instant Pot to pressure cook on high for 5 minutes. Let the pressure release naturally for 5 minutes, then quick-release the steam valve. Add the miso paste and black pepper and stir well to dissolve. Serve immediately.

Leftovers Tip: Store the broth and pasta separately for up to 4 days. Warm the broth on the stovetop until heated through and add the pasta just before serving to avoid mushy noodles.

Per serving: Calories: 645; Fat: 7g; Carbohydrates: 123g; Protein: 22g; Fiber: 12g; Sodium: 927mg

SPICY BUTTERNUT SQUASH BISQUE

GLUTEN-FREE, NUT-FREE

PREP TIME: 10 minutes / **COOK TIME:** 30 minutes / **MAKES 4 SERVINGS**

Since switching to a plant-based diet, I have discovered a love for creamy dishes, and I'm often surprised at the rich texture that can be achieved without any dairy. Take this sweet, silky-smooth butternut squash bisque: it's extremely thick, creamy, and decadent. I suggest adding Crispy Baked Chickpeas (page 146) and pepitas to bump up the protein content and give the soup some textural contrast. This recipe is nice served with a slice of crusty, warm bread for dipping.

Olive oil cooking spray

1 large butternut squash, peeled, seeded and cut into 1-inch cubes (about 3 cups)

2 garlic cloves, peeled

1 teaspoon smoked paprika

½ teaspoon salt

4 cups unsweetened plant-based milk

2 tablespoons nutritional yeast

2 tablespoons tomato paste

1 teaspoon sriracha

4 tablespoons chopped cilantro leaves, for garnish

4 tablespoons plain plant-based yogurt, for garnish

4 tablespoons pepitas, for garnish (optional)

4 tablespoons Crispy Baked Chickpeas (page 146), for garnish (optional)

1. Preheat the oven to 400°F. Spray a sheet pan with olive oil cooking spray.

2. Combine the squash, garlic, smoked paprika, and salt on the sheet pan and toss until evenly coated. Bake for 10 minutes. Using a spatula, turn the squash and continue to bake for another 10 minutes, or until cooked through.

3. Transfer the squash and garlic to a blender. Add the plant-based milk, nutritional yeast, tomato paste, and sriracha and puree until smooth and creamy. Pour the mixture into a large saucepan and cook over medium heat until warm. Taste and adjust the seasonings, if desired.

4. Portion the soup into 4 bowls, garnish each with 1 tablespoon each of cilantro, yogurt, pepitas, and crispy chickpeas (if using), and serve.

Ingredient Tip: You can use 2 (16-ounce) bags of frozen butternut squash instead of fresh and follow the recipe as instructed. No need to thaw.

Per serving (1¾ cups): Calories: 141; Fat: 3g; Carbohydrates: 24g; Protein: 8g; Fiber: 3g; Sodium: 434mg

CHICKPEA CURRY SALAD SANDWICHES

NO COOK, NUT-FREE, ONE BOWL, QUICK, SOY-FREE

PREP TIME: 10 minutes / **MAKES 2 SANDWICHES**

I got the idea for this chickpea salad from a tiny, hole-in-the-wall café that I cheffed at in Emeryville, California, back in the '90s. Curry chicken salad was one of our most popular sandwiches. It is zippy, tangy, crunchy, and slightly sweet. Top these sandwiches with your favorite fixings or forgo the bread and serve the filling mixed into a bowl of greens, tomato, cucumber, and cabbage with a few extra squeezes of lemon.

1 (15-ounce) can chickpeas, drained and rinsed

2 teaspoons store-bought plant-based mayonnaise or Plant-Based Mayo (page 178)

1 apple (any type), cored and chopped in small cubes

Juice of ½ lemon

1 celery stalk, finely chopped

½ cup raisins

1 teaspoon curry powder

¼ teaspoon salt

4 slices whole-wheat bread

1. In a large bowl, mash the chickpeas with the back of a fork. They will break into pieces and get crumbly but not mushy. Add the mayo and mix until well combined.

2. Add the apple, lemon juice, celery, raisins, curry powder, and salt and mix well. Taste and adjust the seasonings, if desired. Sandwich about ¼ cup of filling between 2 slices of bread.

Leftovers Tip: Refrigerate the leftover filling for up to 3 days.

Variation Tip: Use 16 ounces of firm tofu, drained and diced small, instead of chickpeas for a smoother, egg-salad-like texture. Add ¼ cup chopped walnuts for a crunchy twist.

Per serving (1 sandwich): Calories: 489; Fat: 7g; Carbohydrates: 94g; Protein: 18g; Fiber: 15g; Sodium: 874mg

TEMPEH AND LENTIL SLOPPY JOES

NUT-FREE

PREP TIME: 5 minutes / **COOK TIME:** 40 minutes / **MAKES 4 SANDWICHES**

Sloppy joes are an American classic, and in this recipe they get a plant-based update. This is the sloppy joe dreams are made of: slightly sweet, a little tangy, and packed with a protein punch. In fact, this is now one of my favorite ways to prepare tempeh.

5 cups water, divided

¾ cup dried brown lentils, rinsed

2 teaspoons extra-virgin olive oil

½ small yellow onion, diced small

2 garlic cloves, minced

1 (8-ounce) package tempeh

1 teaspoon smoked paprika

3 tablespoons store-bought ketchup or Sugar-Free Ketchup (page 180)

1 tablespoon molasses

1 tablespoon apple cider vinegar

1 teaspoon nutritional yeast

1 teaspoon salt

4 whole-wheat burger buns

1. In a large saucepan, bring 4 cups of water to a boil over high heat. Add the lentils and cook until soft, about 25 minutes. Drain and set aside.

2. In a medium saucepan, heat the oil over medium heat. Add the onion and garlic and cook until browned, 5 to 8 minutes. In a blender or food processor, pulse the tempeh into small pieces.

3. Add the tempeh to the pan with the onion and cook, stirring often, for 2 to 3 minutes. Add the lentils, smoked paprika, ketchup, molasses, apple cider vinegar, nutritional yeast, salt, and the remaining 1 cup water. Simmer, stirring often, until the mixture thickens, about 5 minutes. Divide the mixture among the buns and serve.

Cooking Tip: To shave 20 minutes cooking time off the recipe, drain and use 1 (15-ounce) can of lentils instead of dried.

Per serving (1 sandwich): Calories: 397; Fat: 9g; Carbohydrates: 58g; Protein: 24g; Fiber: 5g; Sodium: 824mg

FETTUCCINE WITH CREAMY CASHEW ALFREDO

PREP TIME: 10 minutes / **COOK TIME:** 30 minutes / **MAKES 4 SERVINGS**

The heavy cheese-and-cream sauce of traditional fettuccine Alfredo never agreed with my constitution, and I learned at a young age that a few moments of palate pleasure were not worth the belly bomb, even though as a budding chef, I was called time and time again to make the dish. Now as a plant-based eater, I have crafted a recipe that is delicious, healthy, and decadent *without* the heaviness of the original.

1 pound whole-grain fettuccine pasta

½ cup frozen peas

2 cups fresh or frozen broccoli florets

1 tablespoon plus 1 teaspoon extra-virgin olive oil, divided

1 cup raw cashews, softened

2 cups water

1 (15-ounce) can cannellini beans, drained and rinsed

1 teaspoon red miso paste

4 garlic cloves, minced

¼ teaspoon onion powder

¼ teaspoon garlic powder

2 tablespoons nutritional yeast

1 teaspoon tapioca flour

2 teaspoons cold water

Salt (optional)

Black pepper

Red pepper flakes, for garnish (optional)

Nutty Plant-Based Parmesan (page 174), for garnish (optional)

1. Bring a large pot of water to a boil over high heat. Add the pasta and cook according to the package instructions. During the last 2 minutes of cook time, add the peas and broccoli. Drain, return to the pot, toss with 1 tablespoon of olive oil to prevent sticking, and set aside.

2. In a blender or food processor, combine the softened cashews, water, beans, and miso paste and blend until smooth. Set aside.

3. In a large saucepan heat the remaining 1 teaspoon olive oil over medium heat. Add the garlic and cook until golden brown and fragrant, about 3 minutes. Add the cashew mixture, onion powder, garlic powder, and the nutritional yeast and stir until combined. Bring to a boil over medium-high heat. Turn the heat to low and let simmer.

4. In a small bowl, make a slurry by whisking together the tapioca flour and cold water. Add the mixture to the saucepan and simmer, stirring constantly, until the sauce thickens, 2 to 3 minutes. Taste and season with salt (if using) and black pepper.

5. Add the sauce to the pot with the pasta and vegetables and toss to coat. To serve, spoon the pasta and vegetables into bowls and garnish with red pepper flakes and plant-based Parmesan (if using).

Cooking Tip: To soften raw cashews, soak them in water overnight and drain and rinse before using. If you're pressed for time, boil them in water for 10 minutes; drain before using.

Leftovers Tip: Store the leftovers for up to 4 days. Reheat in a skillet over low heat with 2 tablespoons unsweetened plant-based milk or water to help loosen and thin out the sauce as it heats.

Per serving: Calories: 741; Fat: 20g; Carbohydrates: 112g; Protein: 33g; Fiber: 18g; Sodium: 144mg

VEGETABLE KORMA CURRY

GLUTEN-FREE, QUICK, SOY-FREE

PREP TIME: 10 minutes / **COOK TIME:** 20 minutes / **MAKES 4 SERVINGS**

Traditional korma dishes use dairy to cook the meat or veggies, which results in a rich curry gravy. My plant-based korma relies on a combo of creamy cashews and coconut milk to braise the potatoes and cauliflower until meltingly tender. The curry is slightly sweet and full of flavor. I suggest serving it over cooked brown rice or quinoa, but cauliflower rice is a great match, too.

1 tablespoon extra-virgin olive oil

2 garlic cloves, minced

2 tablespoons minced
  fresh ginger

½ small yellow onion, diced small

1 medium sweet potato,
  peeled and cut into
  small cubes

½ head cauliflower, cut into small
  florets (about 2 cups)

3 medium tomatoes, diced small

Pinch salt

2 cups water, divided

1 cup softened cashews
  (see Cooking Tip, page 67)

1 tablespoon curry powder

2 tablespoons tomato paste

½ cup frozen green beans

½ cup frozen peas

1 (15-ounce) can light unsweetened coconut milk

2 cups cooked brown rice
  or quinoa, for serving

Chopped fresh cilantro,
  for garnish

Black pepper

1. In a large sauté pan, heat the oil over medium heat. Add the garlic, ginger, and onion and cook until browned and fragrant, about 5 minutes. Add the sweet potato, cauliflower, tomatoes, and salt and cook until the tomatoes begin to break down, about 5 minutes. Add 1 cup of water, stir until combined, and bring the mixture to a boil. Cook until the sweet potatoes are soft, about 10 minutes.

2. In a blender or food processor, combine the cashews with the remaining 1 cup water and blend until you have a smooth paste.

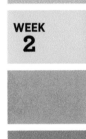

3. Add the blended cashews, curry powder, tomato paste, green beans, peas, and coconut milk to the pan and stir well to combine. Lower the heat to medium-low and simmer for 5 minutes. Taste and adjust the seasoning as desired.

4. Put ½ cup of rice into each serving bowl and top with the curry. Sprinkle with fresh cilantro and black pepper.

Leftovers Tip: Refrigerate the rice topped with the curry for up to 4 days. Microwave in 2-minute increments until heated through.

Per serving: Calories: 535; Fat: 29g; Carbohydrates: 55g; Protein: 14g; Fiber: 8g; Sodium: 69mg

ROASTED CAULIFLOWER BOWLS WITH SPICY GARLIC-TAHINI SAUCE

GLUTEN-FREE, NUT-FREE, QUICK, SOY-FREE

PREP TIME: 10 minutes / **COOK TIME:** 20 minutes / **MAKES 2 SERVINGS**

Nowadays cauliflower is revered for its versatility, low calorie content, and neutral flavor profile. I love roasting it, which imparts a nice smoky flavor, is a low-maintenance cooking method, and gives the cauliflower a pleasant texture that is slightly crisp on the outside and soft on the inside. This cauliflower bowl is easy to execute, and it's bursting with vitamins and Mediterranean flavors. The spicy tahini sauce is to die for.

FOR THE CAULIFLOWER

½ head cauliflower, cut into florets (about 2 cups)

1 tablespoon extra-virgin olive oil

¼ teaspoon black pepper

Juice of ½ lemon

½ teaspoon smoked paprika

1 tablespoon nutritional yeast

½ teaspoon salt

FOR THE GARLIC-TAHINI SAUCE

1 jalapeño pepper, seeded

3 tablespoons tahini

2 garlic cloves

Juice of 1 lemon

½ teaspoon salt

3 tablespoons chopped cilantro

½ cup water

FOR SERVING

2 cups arugula leaves (about 2 ounces)

1 red bell pepper, seeded and thinly sliced

10 kalamata olives, chopped

1 Persian cucumber, sliced

2 tablespoons sesame seeds

1 cup cooked brown rice

1. **Make the cauliflower:** Preheat the oven to 425°F.

2. In a large bowl, mix together the cauliflower florets, olive oil, black pepper, lemon juice, smoked paprika, nutritional yeast, and salt until evenly coated. Spread out the cauliflower in one layer on a sheet pan and bake for 10 minutes. Using a spatula, turn the cauliflower and continue to bake for another 10 minutes.

3. **Make the garlic-tahini sauce:** While the cauliflower is roasting, combine the jalapeño, tahini, garlic, lemon juice, salt, cilantro, and water in a blender and blend until smooth and creamy. Transfer the sauce to a small bowl, cover, and refrigerate until needed.

4. **When ready to serve:** Divide the arugula between 2 plates. Top each evenly with the bell pepper, olives, and cucumbers. Top with the cauliflower and serve with ½ cup of brown rice on the side. Sprinkle with sesame seeds and drizzle with the sauce.

Ingredient Tip: Always inspect cauliflower for black spots and use a knife to remove any. To quickly floret it: first cut the head directly down the center, which exposes the stem that connects all the pieces. Cut out the stem in a triangle shape into the heart of the cauliflower and you will have large florets that can be split into 2 or 3 pieces.

Per serving: Calories: 439; Fat: 27g; Carbohydrates: 43g; Protein: 11g; Fiber: 9g; Sodium: 1,435mg

TEMPEH AND WALNUT "CHORIZO" TACOS

GLUTEN-FREE, QUICK

PREP TIME: 5 minutes / **COOK TIME:** 20 minutes / **MAKES 4 SERVINGS**

In my recipe development process, I accidentally struck gold with this combination of flavors that is undeniably chorizo-like in taste and texture. The mildly nutty tempeh and walnuts grind up nicely in the blender, creating a texture just like the spicy Mexican sausage, and when I added in the smoky spices, it became apparent that this was the real deal. Roll up the mixture in a soft corn tortilla or load it into a crunchy taco with some crispy lettuce, zingy cilantro, and your favorite salsa and you will be *muy feliz.*

- 1 (8-ounce) package tempeh
- 1 cup walnuts
- 1 tablespoon extra-virgin olive oil
- 2 garlic cloves, minced
- 1 small yellow onion, diced very small
- 2 teaspoons tomato paste
- ¼ teaspoon cayenne pepper
- 1½ teaspoons smoked paprika
- 1 teaspoon chili powder
- 1 teaspoon salt
- 1½ cups water
- 12 (6-inch) corn tortillas
- 1 head iceberg lettuce, shredded
- 1 cup chopped fresh cilantro stems and leaves
- 1 cup store-bought salsa or Pico de Gallo (page 172)

1. In a blender, combine the tempeh and walnuts and blend until broken into small pieces resembling ground beef in texture. Set aside.

2. In a large saucepan, heat the olive oil over medium heat. Add the garlic and onion and cook until fragrant, 3 to 5 minutes. Add the tempeh-walnut mixture and cook, stirring often, for 2 to 3 minutes. Add the tomato paste, cayenne, smoked paprika, chili powder, salt, and water, stir until combined, and bring to a boil. Cook, stirring often, until slightly thickened and saucy, about 10 minutes. Remove from the heat.

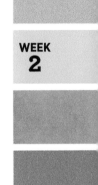

3. In a large skillet, warm the tortillas over medium-high heat, about 2 minutes on each side. Fill the tortillas with equal amounts of filling, lettuce, cilantro, and salsa.

Variation Tip: Substitute 4 ounces of button mushrooms, chopped small, for the walnuts. All the other steps will be the same.

Per serving (3 tacos): Calories: 520; Fat: 30g; Carbohydrates: 53g; Protein: 19g; Fiber: 10g; Sodium: 865mg

CHOCOLATE TAHINI MUFFINS

NUT-FREE, QUICK

PREP TIME: 10 minutes / **COOK TIME:** 20 minutes / **MAKES 12 MUFFINS**

The tahini is what makes these muffins so moist—without the need for any butter or milk. They have just a hint of sweetness from the cocoa powder but are free of refined sugars and full of healthy fats, making them just as appropriate for breakfast as for dessert. Cooking starts with a blast of high heat before you lower the temperature of the oven, yielding a deliciously fluffy final product. Cut one in half and drizzle with some nut butter for an extra energy boost in the morning, or if you are a major chocolate lover, add ½ cup refined-sugar-free chocolate-chunks to the batter.

½ teaspoon, plus 2 tablespoons coconut oil, divided

2 tablespoons ground flaxseeds

6 tablespoons cold water

2 tablespoons tahini

2 tablespoons plain plant-based yogurt

1½ cups unsweetened plant-based milk

2 teaspoons baking powder

½ cup maple syrup

¼ cup unsweetened cocoa powder

½ teaspoon salt

2½ cups whole-wheat flour

1. Preheat the oven to 375°F. Lightly oil a 12-cup muffin tin with ½ tablespoon of coconut oil.

2. In a large bowl, mix together the flaxseed and cold water to make 2 "flax eggs." Let sit for 10 minutes.

3. In a microwave-safe bowl, microwave the remaining 2 tablespoons coconut oil until melted, about 35 seconds. Be careful when removing the bowl so as not to splash hot coconut oil.

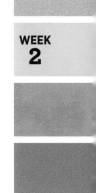

4. Add the coconut oil, tahini, yogurt, plant-based milk, baking powder, and maple syrup to the bowl with the flax eggs and mix well with a fork. Add the cocoa powder, salt, and flour and mix until combined.

5. Divide the batter evenly among the 12 muffin cups, filling each about three-fourths full. Put the muffin pan in the oven and lower the heat to 350°F. Bake for 20 minutes, until a toothpick inserted in the middle comes out clean.

Leftovers Tip: Refrigerate baked muffins for up to 4 days, or refrigerate the batter for up to 3 days and bake a few muffins at a time.

Per serving (1 muffin): Calories: 187; Fat: 6g; Carbohydrates: 31g; Protein: 5g; Fiber: 4g; Sodium: 120mg

Peaches and Cream
Overnight Oats,
page 82

CHAPTER SIX

MEAL PLAN FOR DAYS 15 TO 21

WEEK 3

	Breakfast	Lunch	Dinner
SUNDAY	Choco-Nut Smoothie (page 81)	Sweet Potato, Kale, and Red Cabbage Salad with Avocado-Lime Dressing (page 85)	Lentil Bolognese (page 96)
MONDAY	Peaches and Cream Overnight Oats (page 82)	*Leftover* Lentil Bolognese	Black and White Bean Chili (page 90)
TUESDAY	Tofu, Mushroom, and Spinach Scramble (page 83)	*Leftover* Black and White Bean Chili	Lemony Quinoa Dinner Salad (page 88)
WEDNESDAY	Chickpea and Mushroom Breakfast Bowls (page 84)	*Leftover* Lemony Quinoa Dinner Salad	White Bean, Butternut Squash, and Kale Soup (page 92)
THURSDAY	*Leftover* Tofu, Mushroom, and Spinach Scramble	Creamy Chickpea and Avocado Salad (page 87)	Portobello Mushroom Burgers with Arugula Pesto (page 94)
FRIDAY	*Leftover* Chickpea and Mushroom Breakfast Bowls	*Leftover* White Bean, Butternut Squash, and Kale Soup	Black Bean and Quinoa Burrito Bowls (page 93)
SATURDAY	Choco-Nut Smoothie (page 81)	*Leftover* Portobello Mushroom Burgers with Arugula Pesto	*Leftover* Black Bean and Quinoa Burrito Bowls

Weekly Dessert
Apple Crisp (page 98)

Ingredients You'll Need

FRESH PRODUCE

Apples (6; about 3 pounds)

Arugula (4 cups; 3 to 4 ounces)

Avocados (4)

Bananas (3)

Bell peppers, red or yellow (5)

Butternut squash (½)

Carrots, large (3)

Celery (1 stalk)

Cherry tomatoes (9 ounces)

Cilantro (1 bunch)

Cucumbers, Persian (2)

Garlic (6 cloves)

Jalapeño pepper (1)

Kale (3 bunches)

Lemons (3)

Limes (3)

Mint (1 small package)

Mushrooms, cremini (8 ounces)

Mushrooms, portobello (4)

Mushrooms, white (8 ounces)

Onion, red, small (½)

Onion, yellow, small (2)

Parsley (1 bunch; about 2 ounces)

Peaches, sliced, fresh or frozen (½ cup)

Red cabbage, shredded (1½ cups, plus more for serving)

Scallions (2)

Spinach, baby (4 cups)

Sweet potatoes, medium (2)

Tomatoes, medium (2)

Zucchini, small (1)

CANNED, BOTTLED, AND JARRED

Black beans, 2 (15-ounce) cans

Cannellini beans, 3 (15-ounce) can

Chickpeas, 3 (15-ounce) cans

Coconut milk, light unsweetened, 1 (15-ounce) can

Maple syrup (about ½ cup)

Peanut butter, natural (¼ cup)

Red miso paste (1 teaspoon)

Salsa (for serving)

Tomatoes, crushed, 2 (28-ounce) cans

Tomato paste (2 tablespoons)

REFRIGERATED OR FROZEN

Cauliflower florets, frozen (1 cup)

Corn, frozen (3 cups)

Milk, plant-based, unsweetened (3 cups)

Peas, frozen (1 cup)

Tofu, extra-firm, 1 (16-ounce) package

Yogurt, plant-based, plain unsweetened (2 tablespoons)

CONTINUED ▶

PANTRY

Almonds, slivered
(¼ cup)

Cocoa powder, unsweetened
(2 teaspoons)

Flour, whole-wheat (1 cup)

Hemp hearts
(2 tablespoons)

Lentils, brown or black, dried (1 cup)

Nutritional yeast
(2 tablespoons)

Oats, rolled (1½ cups)

Olives, kalamata (16)

Pasta, whole-wheat, any shape (1 pound)

Pepitas (¼ cup)

Quinoa, dried (1¼ cups)

OTHER

Burger buns, whole-wheat (4)

Staples to Check For: Apple cider vinegar, black pepper, chili powder, coconut oil, extra-virgin olive oil, garlic powder, ground cinnamon, ground cumin, ground turmeric, Italian seasoning, low-sodium soy sauce or gluten-free tamari, onion powder, red pepper flakes, salt, smoked paprika, vanilla extract

Prep This

- Sunday: Prepare the Peaches and Cream Overnight Oats (page 82) for breakfast Monday
- One batch Tangy Cabbage and Kale Slaw (page 144) for the Black Bean and Quinoa Burrito Bowls (page 93) for Friday's dinner (optional)

CHOCO-NUT SMOOTHIE

GLUTEN-FREE, NO COOK, OIL-FREE, QUICK

PREP TIME: 10 minutes / **MAKES 2 SERVINGS**

Smoothies are the ultimate breakfast treat. They are super quick and easy, plus when done right, they can be über-filling. This one utilizes the protein power of peanut butter, the fiber of cauliflower, and the antioxidant-filled decadence of cocoa. Peanut butter and chocolate are a match made in heaven and are the dominant flavors in this addictive morning indulgence.

3 sliced bananas, frozen

3 cups plain unsweetened plant-based milk

¼ cup natural peanut butter

2 teaspoons unsweetened cocoa powder

2 teaspoons maple syrup

1 cup frozen cauliflower florets

In a blender, combine the bananas, plant-based milk, peanut butter, cocoa powder, maple syrup, and cauliflower and puree until smooth.

Variation Tip: For those with peanut allergies, any nut butter will work in this recipe. If all nuts are a no-no, try sunflower seed butter, which is a great alternative.

Per serving: Calories: 583; Fat: 24g; Carbohydrates: 79g; Protein: 23g; Fiber: 10g; Sodium: 210mg

PEACHES AND CREAM OVERNIGHT OATS

NO COOK, OIL-FREE, ONE BOWL

PREP TIME: 10 minutes, plus overnight to chill

MAKES 2 SERVINGS

I don't know what took me so long to jump on the overnight-oats bandwagon, but it's been a game changer. Chilled oats may sound strange, but you have never tasted a creamier and more silky bowl of oats in your life. This breakfast will be your new fave, for both its decadent feel and the convenience of having your breakfast ready and waiting for you in the morning.

½ cup rolled oats

1 cup light unsweetened coconut milk

½ cup peaches, fresh or frozen, diced into 1-inch pieces

½ teaspoon vanilla extract

1 tablespoon maple syrup

Pinch salt

2 tablespoons slivered almonds, for serving

2 tablespoons plain plant-based yogurt, for serving

1. In a medium bowl, mix together the oats, coconut milk, peaches, vanilla, maple syrup, and salt. Cover and refrigerate overnight.

2. To serve, top each serving with 1 tablespoon of slivered almonds and 1 tablespoon of plant-based yogurt.

Ingredients Tip: Refrigerate leftover coconut milk for up to 4 days.

Variation Tip: This luscious overnight oat recipe will work well with any stone fruit or berry. In a pinch, a tablespoon of jam or jelly will give it that same delicious fruity appeal.

Per serving: Calories: 280; Fat: 17g; Carbohydrates: 27g; Protein: 7g; Fiber: 4g; Sodium: 97mg

TOFU, MUSHROOM, AND SPINACH SCRAMBLE

GLUTEN-FREE, NUT-FREE, ONE PAN, QUICK

PREP TIME: 10 minutes / **COOK TIME:** 20 minutes / **MAKES 4 SERVINGS**

A great tofu scramble recipe is worth its weight in gold, and I think this is the only one you'll ever need. The key is to completely sear the tofu in the hot pan, which ensures great texture. This scramble goes well with toasted bread or corn tortillas, or you can roll it into a large flour tortilla and have a breakfast burrito.

1 tablespoon extra-virgin olive oil

1 (16-ounce) package extra-firm tofu, drained and crumbled

½ teaspoon smoked paprika

½ teaspoon ground turmeric

8 ounces white button mushrooms, thinly sliced

2 medium tomatoes, cut into ½-inch dice

4 cups baby spinach

1 scallion, white and green parts, thinly sliced

1 tablespoon low-sodium soy sauce or gluten-free tamari

1. In a large sauté pan, heat the olive oil over medium heat. Add the tofu, smoked paprika, and turmeric and cook without stirring until the tofu is browned, about 5 minutes.

2. Stir the tofu and push it to one side of the pan. Add the mushrooms to the empty side and cook, stirring occasionally, for 5 minutes. Stir the tofu and mushrooms together.

3. Add the tomatoes and cook until they begin to release their juices, 2 to 3 minutes. Add the baby spinach, scallion, and soy sauce and cook, stirring well, until the spinach is wilted. Spoon into 4 bowls and serve. Refrigerate for up to 4 days.

Variation Tip: Try adding 1 chopped zucchini, 1 cup of frozen green peas, or 1 seeded and chopped jalapeño pepper and 1 cup of frozen corn.

Per serving: Calories: 169; Fat: 10g; Carbohydrates: 8g; Protein: 15g; Fiber: 3g; Sodium: 167mg

CHICKPEA AND MUSHROOM BREAKFAST BOWLS

NUT-FREE, ONE PAN, QUICK

PREP TIME: 5 minutes / **COOK TIME:** 15 minutes / **MAKES 4 SERVINGS**

When I discovered that breakfast did not have to be a predictable array of toasted things, sweet stuff, or scrambles it was truly liberating. This breakfast bowl is one of my favorites. It is both light and hearty, super savory, and packs a lot of plant-based protein. The bonus? It comes together in a flash!

1 tablespoon extra-virgin olive oil

1 red or yellow bell pepper, seeded and diced small

8 ounces cremini or white mushrooms, cut into ½-inch-thick slices

1 tablespoon low-sodium soy sauce or gluten-free tamari

½ teaspoon garlic powder

½ teaspoon smoked paprika

1 (15-ounce) can chickpeas, drained and rinsed

1 bunch kale, stemmed and chopped

1 cup frozen peas

2 tablespoons water

1. In a large saucepan, heat the oil over medium heat. Add the bell pepper and mushrooms and cook, stirring occasionally, until the mushrooms are browned, 4 to 5 minutes.

2. Add the soy sauce, garlic powder, smoked paprika, chickpeas, kale, peas, and water and cook until the kale is wilted and fork-tender, about 5 minutes.

Variation Tip: This breakfast can do double duty as a hearty dinner by serving it over 1 cup of leftover cooked grains like quinoa or brown rice.

Per serving: Calories: 205; Fat: 6g; Carbohydrates: 30g; Protein: 12g; Fiber: 9g; Sodium: 321mg

SWEET POTATO, KALE, AND RED CABBAGE SALAD WITH AVOCADO-LIME DRESSING

GLUTEN-FREE, NUT-FREE, QUICK, SOY-FREE

PREP TIME: 10 minutes / **COOK TIME:** 20 minutes / **MAKES 2 SERVINGS**

This salad has such perfectly balanced flavors. The sweetness of the corn and roasted sweet potatoes, the creaminess of avocado, the crunchy pumpkin seeds, and the hardiness of the kale and cabbage is all complemented by a punch of lime and cilantro. It stores very well for leftovers and is easy-peasy to execute.

FOR THE SALAD

1 teaspoon extra-virgin olive oil

2 medium sweet potatoes, peeled and diced small

Pinch salt

1 cup frozen corn

2 cups stemmed and chopped kale

1 cup shredded red cabbage

¼ cup pepitas

FOR THE DRESSING

1 avocado, peeled and pitted

Juice of 1½ limes

Pinch salt

Pinch red pepper flakes (optional)

3 tablespoons chopped fresh cilantro leaves

½ cup water

1. **Make the salad:** Preheat the oven to 425°F. Grease a sheet pan with the olive oil.

2. Spread the sweet potato on the prepared sheet pan in one layer and sprinkle with salt. Bake for 10 minutes. Using a spatula, turn the potatoes and continue to bake for another 5 minutes. Add the corn to the sheet pan and bake everything for 5 minutes more.

CONTINUED ▶

3. **Make the dressing:** In a blender, combine the avocado, lime juice, salt, red pepper flakes (if using), cilantro, and water and blend until smooth.

4. **Assemble the salad:** In a large bowl, combine the kale and cabbage, add half of the dressing, and toss gently. Add the sweet potatoes, corn, and the remaining dressing and toss until combined. The warm corn and sweet potatoes will help soften the kale slightly. Divide the salad between 2 bowls, top with the pepitas, and serve.

Leftovers Tip: Normally, I would advise storing salads and dressings separately, but kale is a hardy green and will be fine with the dressing. In fact, it will taste even better the next day. Just be sure to refrigerate it and eat it within 3 days for best results.

Per serving: Calories: 488; Fat: 25g; Carbohydrates: 64g; Protein: 13g; Fiber: 16g; Sodium: 296mg

CREAMY CHICKPEA AND AVOCADO SALAD

GLUTEN-FREE, NO COOK, OIL-FREE, ONE PAN, QUICK, SOY-FREE

PREP TIME: 20 minutes / **MAKES 2 SERVINGS**

Tuna salad was a staple in my childhood lunches, and I think this chickpea version is even tastier. I love its fresh Mediterranean flavors, and the avocado makes it extra creamy and delicious without added oils or mayonnaise. You can eat this straight out of the bowl, perch it atop a bed of salad greens, or use it as filling in a sandwich or wrap.

WEEK 3

- 1 (15-ounce) can chickpeas, drained and rinsed
- 1 avocado, peeled and pitted
- 2 tablespoons slivered almonds
- 1 celery stalk, minced
- 1 large carrot, peeled and grated or minced
- 3 cherry tomatoes, diced small
- 6 kalamata olives, pitted and chopped
- Juice of 1 lemon
- 2 tablespoons chopped fresh parsley
- ½ teaspoon salt

1. In a medium bowl, combine the chickpeas and avocados and mash with a fork, until the avocado is smooth and the chickpeas are mostly broken but still chunky.

2. Add the almonds, celery, carrot, tomatoes, olives, lemon juice, parsley, and salt and mix until well combined. Serve immediately.

Variation Tip: Switch up the flavor profile by subbing in dill for the parsley, skipping the olives, and adding 1 chopped Persian cucumber.

Per serving: Calories: 396; Fat: 22g; Carbohydrates: 43g; Protein: 12g; Fiber: 17g; Sodium: 991mg

LEMONY QUINOA DINNER SALAD

GLUTEN-FREE, NUT-FREE, QUICK

PREP TIME: 10 minutes / **COOK TIME:** 20 minutes / **MAKES 4 SERVINGS**

This main-course salad was inspired by a visit to Greece, where I fell in love with their fresh lemon- and herb-infused cooking. While quinoa may not be quintessentially Greek, it does lend itself well to the Mediterranean flavors and gives a great heartiness and protein punch to this seemingly light dish. I could eat this one every day.

⅔ cup quinoa

2½ tablespoons extra-virgin olive oil, divided

Pinch plus ½ teaspoon salt, divided

2 Persian cucumbers, diced small

8 ounces cherry tomatoes, halved

10 kalamata olives, pitted and chopped

6 mint leaves, chopped

3 tablespoons chopped fresh parsley

1 (15-ounce) can chickpeas, drained and rinsed

½ red onion, diced small

½ cup shredded red cabbage

Juice of 1 lemon, plus more for serving

1 tablespoon apple cider vinegar

1 teaspoon maple syrup

1 teaspoon Italian seasoning

Pinch red pepper flakes

Pinch black pepper, plus more for serving

2 cups arugula

1. Cook the quinoa according to the package instructions, adding ½ tablespoon olive oil and a pinch of salt with the quinoa.

2. In a large bowl, mix together the cucumbers, cherry tomatoes, olives, mint, parsley, chickpeas, onions, and cabbage. Set aside.

3. In a small bowl, whisk together the lemon juice, apple cider vinegar, maple syrup, the remaining ½ teaspoon salt, the Italian seasoning, red pepper flakes, and black pepper. Pour the mixture over the vegetables and toss until evenly coated.

4. To serve, divide the arugula among 4 bowls. Top each portion with a quarter of the chopped salad mix and a quarter of the cooked quinoa. Serve with a squeeze of lemon juice and a sprinkle of black pepper.

Leftovers Tip: Toss the quinoa and vegetable mixture with the dressing and refrigerate for up to 3 days. The quinoa will absorb the dressing and will be a perfect leftover lunch on the bed of arugula; store the arugula separately so that it doesn't wilt.

Calories: 268; Fat: 13g; Carbohydrates: 32g; Protein: 8g; Fiber: 7g; Sodium: 534mg

BLACK AND WHITE BEAN CHILI

GLUTEN-FREE, NUT-FREE, ONE POT, QUICK, SOY-FREE

PREP TIME: 10 minutes / **COOK TIME:** 20 minutes / **MAKES 4 SERVINGS**

Veggie chili has been a staple in my diet for many years. Even when I was an omnivore, I always left out the meat because it tastes so good without it. This chili is chock-full of beans and vegetables, and instead of drowning out all the flavors with a heavy chili powder, I spice it just enough to make those ingredients pop! The corn is sweet and the sauce is tangy, and I guarantee you will not miss the meat. Feel free to serve with soft corn tortillas on the side.

1 teaspoon extra-virgin olive oil

½ yellow onion, diced small

1 large carrot, peeled and
   diced small

1 red or yellow bell pepper,
   seeded and diced small

1 small zucchini, diced small

1 (15-ounce) can cannellini beans,
   drained and rinsed

1 (15-ounce) can black beans,
   drained and rinsed

1 (28-ounce) can crushed
   tomatoes

1 cup frozen corn

1 teaspoon chili powder

½ teaspoon salt

½ teaspoon ground cumin

½ teaspoon garlic powder

1 cup water

2 tablespoons minced fresh
   cilantro, for garnish

Pinch red pepper flakes,
   for garnish

1 scallion, white and green parts,
   thinly sliced, for garnish

1 jalapeño pepper, cut into slices,
   for garnish (optional)

1 avocado, peeled, pitted,
   and diced, for garnish

1 lime, cut into wedges,
   for garnish

1. In a large pot, heat the olive oil over medium heat. Add the onion, carrot, bell pepper, and zucchini and cook, stirring often, until fragrant and the vegetables start to get tender, about 10 minutes.

2. Raise the heat to medium-high, add the cannellini beans, black beans, tomatoes, corn, chili powder, salt, cumin, garlic powder, and water, stir well, and bring to a boil. Lower the heat to medium-low and simmer until heated through and the flavors meld, about 5 more minutes.

3. Spoon the chili into bowls and garnish with cilantro, red pepper flakes, scallion, jalapeño (if using), avocado, and a lime wedge.

Variation Tip: For a smoother, saucier chili, combine the onion, carrot, bell pepper, and zucchini in the blender first to almost puree them before cooking them in the oil.

Per serving: Calories: 329; Fat: 3g; Carbohydrates: 65g; Protein: 17g; Fiber: 20g; Sodium: 699mg

WHITE BEAN, BUTTERNUT SQUASH, AND KALE SOUP

GLUTEN-FREE, NUT-FREE, QUICK

PREP TIME: 15 minutes / **COOK TIME:** 15 minutes / **MAKES 4 SERVINGS**

This soup is astoundingly easy and deliciously creamy. The miso fortifies the soup with a deep umami flavor.

½ medium butternut squash, peeled, seeded, and cut into small pieces (about 2 cups)

4 cups water, divided

1 bunch kale, stemmed, leaves chopped small

2 (15-ounce) cans cannellini beans, drained and rinsed

1½ teaspoons salt

1½ teaspoons onion powder

1 teaspoon garlic powder

½ teaspoon smoked paprika

1 teaspoon red miso paste

Red pepper flakes

1. In a medium saucepan combine the squash with 2 cups of water and bring to a boil over high heat. Lower the heat to medium and cook until it is fork-tender, about 5 minutes.

2. Using a slotted spoon, transfer half of the softened squash to a blender with the remaining 2 cups water and blend until smooth. Add it back to the pot.

3. Add the kale, cannellini beans, salt, onion powder, garlic powder, and smoked paprika and bring to a boil. Cook until the kale is tender, about 5 minutes.

4. Remove from the heat, add the miso, and stir well until the miso dissolves. Spoon into bowls and sprinkle with red pepper flakes.

Per serving (2½ cups): Calories: 273; Fat: 2g; Carbohydrates: 53g; Protein: 16g; Fiber: 19g; Sodium: 961mg

BLACK BEAN AND QUINOA BURRITO BOWLS

GLUTEN-FREE, NUT-FREE, QUICK, SOY-FREE

PREP TIME: 10 minutes / **COOK TIME:** 10 minutes / **MAKES 4 SERVINGS**

The combo of black beans and quinoa is a nutritional match made in heaven. The powerful plant-based protein plus the high fiber count will keep you full for hours.

WEEK 3

1 cup quinoa

1 cup frozen corn

1 teaspoon extra-virgin olive oil

1 tablespoon tomato paste

½ teaspoon salt, divided

2¼ cups water

1 (15-ounce) can black beans

½ teaspoon onion powder

½ teaspoon garlic powder

1 avocado, peeled, pitted, and sliced, for serving

Shredded red cabbage or Tangy Cabbage and Kale Slaw (page 144), for serving

Store-bought salsa or Pico de Gallo (page 172), for serving

¼ cup chopped fresh cilantro, for garnish

1. In a medium saucepan over medium-high heat, combine the quinoa, corn, oil, tomato paste, ¼ teaspoon of salt, and the water and bring it to a boil. Cover, lower the heat to low, and cook until the quinoa is tender and the water is absorbed, about 15 minutes.

2. In a skillet over medium heat, combine the black beans, onion powder, garlic powder, and the remaining ¼ teaspoon salt and cook, stirring, for 5 minutes.

3. To assemble, divide the quinoa mixture, black beans, avocado, cabbage, and salsa among 4 bowls. Garnish with the cilantro.

Variation Tip: Substitute brown rice or riced cauliflower for the quinoa. You can make your own cauli rice by grating a head of cauliflower on the biggest holes of a box grater and lightly steaming it.

Per serving: Calories: 378; Fat: 12g; Carbohydrates: 58g; Protein: 14g; Fiber: 13g; Sodium: 302mg

PORTOBELLO MUSHROOM BURGERS WITH ARUGULA PESTO

NUT-FREE, QUICK, SOY-FREE

PREP TIME: 10 minutes / **COOK TIME:** 20 minutes / **MAKES 4 BURGERS**

Most people either love or hate mushrooms. I am of the love school, and these slightly crispy, smoky, seasoned portobellos are heavenly on a bun with my famous arugula pesto. Portobellos are the "meat" of the fungus world, full of B vitamins and antioxidants. You will love them, too, and the nut-free pesto is sure to be a favorite.

---

5 teaspoons extra-virgin olive oil, divided

1 teaspoon smoked paprika

1 teaspoon garlic powder

1 teaspoon salt, divided

4 portobello mushroom caps

2 cups arugula

2 garlic cloves, peeled

Juice of ½ lemon

2 tablespoons hemp hearts

2 tablespoons nutritional yeast

1 small yellow onion, cut into ¼-inch slices

2 red or yellow bell peppers, seeded and cut into quarters

4 whole-wheat burger buns, for serving

Shredded red cabbage, for serving (optional)

1. In a large bowl, mix together 2 teaspoons of olive oil, the smoked paprika, garlic powder, and ½ teaspoon of salt. Add the portobellos and gently turn to coat them well with the seasonings.

2. In a blender, combine the arugula, garlic, lemon juice, hemp hearts, nutritional yeast, 1 teaspoon of olive oil, and the remaining ½ teaspoon salt and blend until smooth. Set aside.

3. In a large skillet, heat 1 teaspoon of olive oil over medium heat. Add the onions and bell peppers and cook, stirring, until the onions are browned and fragrant, about 10 minutes

4. At the same time, in a large skillet over medium heat, pour in the remaining 1 teaspoon oil. Add the mushrooms, gill-side down, and place another pan or heat-safe plate on top of the mushrooms to weigh them down. This will help sear the mushrooms and give them a better texture. Cook for 5 minutes, flip the mushrooms, replace the weight on the mushrooms, and cook 5 more minutes.

5. For each burger, spread 1 tablespoon of arugula pesto onto each bun. Top with 1 portobello, a quarter of the bell pepper, a quarter of the caramelized onions, and red cabbage (if using).

> **Leftovers Tip:** Store the leftover mushrooms separate from the buns and toppings. Simply reheat them in a skillet for the next meal. Fill an airtight container with left-over pesto, and cover the top with olive oil to preserve the color. It will last up to a week in the refrigerator or 3 months in the freezer.

Per serving (1 burger): Calories: 244; Fat: 9g; Carbohydrates: 33g; Protein: 13g; Fiber: 4g; Sodium: 806mg

LENTIL BOLOGNESE

NUT-FREE, SOY-FREE

PREP TIME: 10 minutes / **COOK TIME:** 30 minutes / **MAKES 4 SERVINGS**

Bolognese, or "meat sauce" as it was called in my home, was always a favorite with the family when I was a kid, and in adulthood it's no different. This plant-based version is delightfully hearty, filling, and delicious. Full of both flavor and nutrients, it is sure to be a winner in your home, too.

---

1 cup dried brown or black lentils, rinsed

3 cups water

1 pound whole-wheat pasta

1 teaspoon extra-virgin olive oil

4 garlic cloves, minced

½ small yellow onion, diced small

1 red or yellow bell pepper, seeded and diced small

1 large carrot, peeled and finely chopped

1 (28-ounce) can crushed tomatoes

2 teaspoons tomato paste

Pinch red pepper flakes

1 teaspoon maple syrup

½ teaspoon Italian seasoning

1 teaspoon salt

Black pepper

2 tablespoons chopped fresh parsley, for garnish

2 tablespoons chopped fresh mint, for garnish

1. In a large saucepan, combine the lentils and water and bring to a boil. Lower the heat to medium-low and cook until soft, about 25 minutes.

2. Bring a large pot of water to a boil over high heat. Add the pasta and cook according to the package instructions. Drain and set aside.

3. In a large saucepan, heat the oil over medium heat. Add the garlic, onion, bell pepper, and carrot and cook, stirring often, until fragrant, 5 to 10 minutes.

4. Add the tomatoes, tomato paste, red pepper flakes, maple syrup, Italian seasoning, and salt, stir until combined, and bring to a boil.

5. Drain the lentils, add them to the tomato sauce, and stir until combined. Add the pasta to the sauce and toss until evenly coated. Serve in shallow bowls, sprinkled with black pepper, parsley, and mint.

Cooking Tip: To reduce the preparation time, use 2 (15-ounce) cans of lentils instead of dried. Drain before adding them to the tomato sauce and cook until heated through.

Per serving: Calories: 547; Fat: 4g; Carbohydrates: 110g; Protein: 21g; Fiber: 9g; Sodium: 1,001mg

APPLE CRISP

NUT-FREE, SOY-FREE

PREP TIME: 15 minutes / **COOK TIME:** 40 minutes / **MAKES 4 SERVINGS**

Apple crisp is truly one of the few desserts that delight me. The heavenly smell as it is baking transports me back to the Thanksgivings of my childhood, when the only care in the world was when I would be allowed to have some dessert. This recipe is so easy, and there is almost no perceptible difference from the butter-filled classic.

6 apples (about 3 pounds), peeled, cored, and chopped

3 teaspoons ground cinnamon, divided

5 tablespoons maple syrup, divided

¼ cup coconut oil, melted

1 cup whole-wheat flour

1 cup rolled oats

1. Preheat the oven to 350°F.

2. In a large bowl, mix together the apples, 2 teaspoons of cinnamon, and 2 tablespoons of maple syrup.

3. In another bowl, mix together the remaining 1 teaspoon cinnamon, remaining 3 tablespoons maple syrup, the coconut oil, flour, and oats until it forms a crumbly dough.

4. Transfer the apple mixture to an 8-by-8-inch baking dish. Crumble the flour-and-oat mixture loosely over the top of the apples. Bake for 40 to 50 minutes, until the topping is crisp and the apples are bubbling.

Leftovers Tip: Refrigerate leftovers for up to 3 days.

Variation Tip: Mix ½ cup of fresh cranberries with the apples and add another tablespoon of maple syrup.

Per serving: Calories: 481; Fat: 16g; Carbohydrates: 84g; Protein: 8g; Fiber: 10g; Sodium: 4mg

Chickpea Coconut
Curry, page 114

CHAPTER SEVEN

MEAL PLAN FOR DAYS 22 TO 30

WEEK 4

	Breakfast	Lunch	Dinner
SUNDAY	Dutch Apple Pie Oatmeal Squares (page 106)	BBQ Tempeh Succotash Skillet (page 120)	White Bean and Kale Linguine (page 117)
MONDAY	Overnight Pumpkin Spice Chia Pudding (page 107)	Warm Lentil Salad with Tomato Vinaigrette (page 112)	Chickpea Coconut Curry (page 114)
TUESDAY	Tofu Rancheros (page 110)	*Leftover* White Bean and Kale Linguine	Pulled Jackfruit Tacos (page 119)
WEDNESDAY	*Leftover* Overnight Pumpkin Spice Chia Pudding	Spiced Eggplant and Hummus Sandwiches (page 115)	Mushroom Barley Soup (page 113)
THURSDAY	Green Goodness Smoothies (page 108)	*Leftover* BBQ Tempeh Succotash Skillet	Meatless Meatballs with Quick Marinara Sauce (page 122)
FRIDAY	Avocado Toast with Tomato and Hemp Hearts (page 109)	*Leftover* Chickpea Coconut Curry	Chickpea, Butternut Squash, and Herb Stuffed Peppers (page 126)
SATURDAY	*Leftover* Tofu Rancheros	*Leftover* Mushroom Barley Soup	Rainbow Shepherd's Pie (page 124)

Weekly Dessert
Chocolate Pudding with Raspberries and Mint (page 128)

Ingredients You'll Need

FRESH PRODUCE

Apple (1)

Arugula (1 cup)

Avocados (5)

Baby bell peppers, sweet (3)

Bananas (3)

Basil (6 leaves)

Bell pepper, green (1)

Bell peppers, red or yellow (9)

Carrots, large (4)

Cauliflower (2 heads)

Celery (1 stalk)

Cilantro (1 small bunch)

Coleslaw mix (for serving)

Collard greens (1 bunch)

Eggplant, Italian (1; ½ pound)

Garlic (18 cloves; about 2 heads)

Ginger (2 inches)

Kale (1 bunch; 3 cups stemmed and chopped)

Lemon (1)

Lime (1)

Mint (1 small package)

Mushrooms, white (8 ounces)

Onion, yellow, small (4)

Parsley (1 small bunch)

Raspberries (16; about ½ cup)

Scallions (4)

Spinach, baby (7 to 8 cups)

Sweet potatoes, medium (4)

Tomatoes, medium (6)

CANNED, BOTTLED, AND JARRED

Barbecue sauce (2 tablespoons)

Black beans, 1 (15-ounce) can

Cannellini beans, 1 (15-ounce) can

Chickpeas, 4 (15-ounce) cans

Coconut milk, full-fat unsweetened, 1 (15-ounce) can

Coconut milk, light unsweetened, 1 (15-ounce) can

Crushed tomatoes, 2 (15-ounce) cans

Crushed tomatoes, 1 (28-ounce) can

Jackfruit, 1 (15-ounce) can

Lentils, 1 (15-ounce) can

Maple syrup (1 cup)

Pumpkin puree, unsweetened, 1 (15-ounce) can

Salsa (for serving)

Tomato paste (about ¼ cup)

WEEK
4

CONTINUED ▶

Meal Plan for Days 22 to 30   **103**

REFRIGERATED OR FROZEN

Brown rice, cooked or frozen (3 cups)

Butternut squash, cubed, frozen (2 cups)

Cauliflower florets, frozen (1 cup)

Corn, frozen (1½ cups)

Guacamole (for serving)

Hummus (¼ cup)

Milk, plant-based, unsweetened (3¼ cups)

Peas, frozen (1 cup)

Tempeh, 2 (8-ounce) packages

Tofu, extra-firm, 2 (16-ounce) packages

Tofu, silken, 1 (16-ounce) package

PANTRY

Balsamic vinegar (2 tablespoons)

Barley, pearled (1 cup)

Chia seeds (¾ cup)

Coconut water (3 cups)

Flaxseeds, ground (about ⅓ cup)

Flour, tapioca (4 teaspoons)

Flour, whole-wheat (½ cup plus 2 tablespoons)

Hemp hearts (4 teaspoons)

Linguine, whole-wheat (1 pound)

Macadamia nuts (¾ cup)

Nutritional yeast (3 tablespoons)

Oats, rolled (3¼ cups)

Olives, kalamata (10)

Pecans (½ cup)

Pumpkin spice blend (1 tablespoon)

Sesame seeds (2 tablespoons, optional)

Split peas, dried (2 cups)

Sunflower seeds (1 tablespoon)

Thyme, dried (¼ teaspoon)

OTHER

Bread, whole-wheat (8 slices)

Tortillas, corn, 6-inch (20)

Staples to Check For: Black pepper, cayenne pepper, chili powder, curry powder, extra-virgin olive oil, garlic powder, ground cinnamon, ground turmeric, Italian seasoning, low-sodium soy sauce or gluten-free tamari, onion powder, red pepper flakes, salt, smoked paprika, unsweetened cocoa powder, vanilla extract

Prep This

- Sunday: Prep the Overnight Pumpkin Spice Chia Pudding (page 107) for Monday breakfast; Freeze 3 bananas for the Green Goodness Smoothies (page 108)

- One batch of Tangy Cabbage and Kale Slaw (page 144) and one batch Super-Simple Guacamole (page 171) for the Pulled Jackfruit Tacos (page 119) for Tuesday's dinner (optional)

- One batch Garlic Hummus (page 147) for the Spiced Eggplant and Hummus Sandwiches (page 115) for Wednesday's lunch (optional)

WEEK
4

DUTCH APPLE PIE OATMEAL SQUARES

OIL-FREE

PREP TIME: 10 minutes / **COOK TIME:** 30 minutes / **MAKES 4 SERVINGS**

There are a few desserts that really float my boat, like Dutch apple pie and apple crumble. I tasked myself with developing a recipe for baked oatmeal that mimics the experience of Dutch apple pie with a soft interior and a crispy and crumbly topping.

2¼ cups rolled oats, divided

1 cup unsweetened plant-based milk

4 tablespoons maple syrup, divided

2 teaspoons ground cinnamon

1 apple, peeled, cored, and chopped

1 teaspoon vanilla extract

¼ cup ground flaxseeds

1 cup plus 3 tablespoons water, divided

¼ cup macadamia nuts

½ cup whole-wheat flour

1. Preheat the oven to 375°F.

2. In an 8-by-8-inch baking dish, mix together 2 cups of oats, the plant-based milk, 2 tablespoons of maple syrup, the cinnamon, apple, vanilla, flaxseeds, and 1 cup of water.

3. In a blender, pulse the macadamia nuts to a meal-like texture.

4. In a medium bowl, mix together the whole-wheat flour, macadamia nuts, the remaining ¼ cup oats, remaining 2 tablespoons maple syrup, and 3 tablespoons water to form a loose dough. Crumble the mixture over the top of the oatmeal mixture.

5. Bake for 35 minutes, or until the top is crispy. Let cool for 10 minutes to set, then cut into 4 squares. Refrigerate for up to 4 days.

Per serving: Calories: 438; Fat: 14g; Carbohydrates: 69g; Protein: 14g; Fiber: 11g; Sodium: 36mg

OVERNIGHT PUMPKIN SPICE CHIA PUDDING

GLUTEN-FREE, NO COOK, OIL-FREE, ONE BOWL

PREP TIME: 10 minutes, plus overnight to chill / **MAKES 4 SERVINGS**

Few things around the holiday season are as revered as pumpkin spice. Here is an easy and delicious way to enjoy this festive flavor all year-round. I combined pumpkin puree with chia seeds, creating a pudding you really need to try. The pumpkin makes it smooth and the chia contributes a texture that is similar to tapioca. Garnish with any kind of nuts you have, but I think pecans are the best flavor combo.

WEEK
4

¾ **cup chia seeds**

2 **cups unsweetened plant-based milk**

1 **(15-ounce) can unsweetened pumpkin puree**

¼ **cup maple syrup**

1 **tablespoon pumpkin pie spice blend**

1 **cup water**

½ **cup pecans, for serving**

1. In a large bowl, whisk together the chia seeds, plant-based milk, pumpkin puree, maple syrup, pumpkin pie spice, and water.

2. Divide the mixture among 4 mason jars or containers with lids. Let sit for 10 minutes. Stir each container to break up any chia clumps. Cover and refrigerate overnight to firm up. To serve, garnish each with some of the pecans.

Variation Tip: If you don't like the texture of tapioca pudding, chances are you might not like the consistency of chia pudding. You can make it more like traditional pudding by putting it into a blender and pureeing until smooth.

Per serving: Calories: 421; Fat: 23g; Carbohydrates: 47g; Protein: 12g; Fiber: 20g; Sodium: 74mg

GREEN GOODNESS SMOOTHIES

GLUTEN-FREE, NUT-FREE, QUICK, NO COOK, OIL-FREE, ONE BOWL

PREP TIME: 5 minutes / **MAKES 2 SERVINGS**

When people think of smoothies, they usually picture a sweet, fruity drink that is pink or orange and full of fluffy ingredients rather than a truly hearty or filling meal. This green smoothie is the quintessential horse of a different color. The bright hue is striking, but even more stunning is the taste. Only slightly sweet, the ingredients balance each other so well, you won't remember that you are getting four servings of produce in one refreshing drinkable meal. You may be shocked at the addition of cauliflower in this smoothie's ingredients, but you won't even notice it!

3 frozen sliced bananas

3 cups coconut water

1 cup baby spinach

1 cup frozen cauliflower florets

2 tablespoons ground flaxseeds

1 avocado, peeled and pitted

2 teaspoons maple syrup, plus
more as needed

In a high-speed blender, combine the bananas, coconut water, spinach, cauliflower, flaxseeds, avocado, and maple syrup and blend until smooth. Taste for sweetness and adjust by adding more maple syrup as needed.

Ingredient Tip: Right after shopping, peel and cut the bananas into 2-inch slices and put them in an airtight container. They can be stored for 2 months in the freezer so you'll always be ready to make smoothies.

Per serving: Calories: 307; Fat: 13g; Carbohydrates: 48g; Protein: 6g; Fiber: 13g; Sodium: 278mg

AVOCADO TOAST WITH TOMATO AND HEMP HEARTS

5 INGREDIENTS, NUT-FREE, QUICK, SOY-FREE

PREP TIME: 5 minutes / **COOK TIME:** 5 minutes / **MAKES 2 SERVINGS**

The first time I heard about avocado toast, I thought the idea was so simple and understated that I had to try it. Ten years later, and avo toast is one of my breakfast staples. There is nothing as perfect as salted and mashed avocado spread atop some whole-wheat toast. It's a quick and easy breakfast that offers a nice, slow burn of energy due to the avocado's healthy fats and the toast's complex carbs. I've added tangy, fresh tomato slices and some superfood hemp hearts to amp up this 10-minute breakfast.

4 slices whole-wheat bread

1 avocado, peeled, pitted, cut into quarters, and thinly sliced

Salt

1 medium tomato, thinly sliced

Black pepper

Red pepper flakes

2 teaspoons extra-virgin olive oil

4 teaspoons hemp hearts

1. Toast the bread slices.

2. On each slice, arrange a quarter of the avocado slices, a pinch of salt, a quarter of the tomato, a pinch of black pepper, and a pinch of red pepper flakes. Drizzle each with ½ teaspoon of olive oil and sprinkle with 1 teaspoon of hemp hearts.

Variation Tip: This simple foundation is easy to build on and is a great way to avoid food waste. The buttery avocado pairs well with mint, basil, cilantro, parsley, or any fresh herb you have on hand. Drizzle with lemon or lime juice. Or try topping it with leftover beans or greens.

Per serving: Calories: 379; Fat: 22g; Carbohydrates: 38g; Protein: 12g; Fiber: 11g; Sodium: 411mg

TOFU RANCHEROS

GLUTEN-FREE, NUT-FREE, QUICK

PREP TIME: 10 minutes / **COOK TIME:** 20 minutes / **MAKES 4 SERVINGS**

Before I had kids, I used to brunch a lot, and huevos rancheros was the thing I always ordered. This plant-based version captures the essence of the original dish while using spiced tofu. Even without eggs or cheese, it is super tasty with the delicious Mexican flavors of salsa, warm tortillas, beans, and avocado.

1 (15-ounce) can black beans, drained and rinsed

½ teaspoon onion powder

½ teaspoon garlic powder

2½ cups water, divided

1 teaspoon extra-virgin olive oil

½ head cauliflower, cut into florets (about 2 cups)

1 red or yellow bell pepper, seeded and diced small

1 (16-ounce) package extra firm-tofu, drained and diced small

½ teaspoon salt, plus more as needed

1 teaspoon smoked paprika

2 medium tomatoes, cut into ½-inch pieces

2 teaspoons tomato paste

1 teaspoon chili powder

2 avocados, peeled and pitted

8 (6-inch) corn tortillas

3 tablespoons chopped fresh cilantro, for serving

2 scallions, white and green parts, thinly sliced, for serving

1 lime, cut into quarters, for serving

1. In a small saucepan over medium heat, combine the beans, onion powder, garlic powder, and ½ cup of water and cook until heated through, 5 to 7 minutes. Set aside.

2. In a large saucepan, heat the oil over medium heat. Add the cauliflower and bell pepper and cook, stirring occasionally, for 2 to 3 minutes. Add the tofu, salt, and smoked paprika and cook, stirring often, for 5 minutes.

3. Add the tomatoes, tomato paste, and chili powder and cook, stirring often, until the tomatoes release their juices and the tomato paste turns dark red, 2 to 3 minutes. Add the remaining 2 cups water, stir well, and bring to a boil. Cook until the sauce is thick and the flavors meld, about 4 minutes.

4. In a small bowl, combine the avocados and a pinch of salt and mash until well mixed.

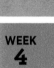

5. In a large skillet, warm the tortillas over medium-high heat, about 2 minutes on each side. Put 2 tortillas on a plate, layer with the tofu mixture, scallions, cilantro, a big dollop of mashed avocado, and a squeeze of lime juice. Put a scoop of black beans on the side and serve.

Ingredient Tip: You can use frozen cauliflower florets. Add them to the recipe at the same time you would the fresh cauliflower and cook as instructed.

Leftovers Tip: Refrigerate all the components separately for up to 4 days. Heat only enough tortillas for serving. The tofu and beans can be reheated in the microwave in 2-minute increments until warmed through.

Per serving: Calories: 590; Fat: 27g; Carbohydrates: 69g; Protein: 27g; Fiber: 18g; Sodium: 783mg

WARM LENTIL SALAD WITH TOMATO VINAIGRETTE

GLUTEN-FREE, NUT-FREE, QUICK, SOY-FREE

PREP TIME: 10 minutes / **COOK TIME:** 15 minutes / **MAKES 2 SERVINGS**

This tasty take on salad was inspired by my days at the Westside Café in Berkeley. The earthy lentils are complemented so well by the garlicky, herbed tomatoes, caramelized balsamic vinegar, and the tangy kalamata olives.

2 teaspoons extra-virgin olive oil

2 garlic cloves, chopped

1 tablespoon Italian seasoning

½ head cauliflower, cut into florets (about 2 cups)

1 large carrot, peeled and diced small

2 medium tomatoes, diced small

10 kalamata olives, pitted and halved

1 teaspoon salt

½ teaspoon black pepper

2 tablespoons balsamic vinegar

1 (15-ounce) can brown lentils

1 cup water

4 cups baby spinach

1 tablespoon sunflower seeds

1. In a large saucepan, heat the olive oil over medium heat. Add the garlic and Italian seasoning and cook until fragrant, 2 to 3 minutes.

2. Add the cauliflower, carrot, tomatoes, olives, salt, and black pepper and cook, stirring often, for 2 to 3 minutes. Add the balsamic vinegar and cook to caramelize the sugars in the vinegar, 2 to 3 minutes.

3. Add the lentils and water, bring to a boil, and cook for 2 to 3 minutes until heated throughout. Remove from the heat.

4. In a large bowl, toss together the spinach and sunflower seeds. Add the lentil mixture and toss until the spinach is wilted.

Ingredient Tip: You can use frozen cauliflower florets, but you may need to increase the cooking time.

Per serving: Calories: 363; Fat: 10g; Carbohydrates: 53g; Protein: 21g; Fiber: 19g; Sodium: 1,503mg

MUSHROOM BARLEY SOUP

NUT-FREE, ONE POT, SOY-FREE

PREP TIME: 10 minutes / **COOK TIME:** 40 minutes / **MAKES 4 SERVINGS**

Barley is an underappreciated grain: it has a formidable protein content, is high in fiber, and is also a great source of iron and magnesium. Plus, its mild flavor works very well with the umami of mushrooms.

1 cup pearled barley

4 cups water

2 teaspoons extra-virgin olive oil, divided

1 small yellow onion, diced small

3 garlic cloves, minced

2 large carrots, peeled and diced small

1 celery stalk, minced

8 ounces white mushrooms, thinly sliced

1 teaspoon salt

¼ teaspoon dried thyme

½ teaspoon smoked paprika

1. In a large pot, combine the barley and water and bring to a boil over high heat. Lower the heat to medium-low and cook until tender, about 40 minutes.

2. While the barley is cooking, in a large skillet, heat 1 teaspoon of olive oil over medium heat. Add the onion, garlic, carrots, and celery and cook, stirring often, until the vegetables are tender, about 8 minutes. Add the mixture to the barley.

3. Wipe out the skillet with a paper towel. Heat the remaining 1 teaspoon oil over medium heat. Add the mushrooms and cook, stirring occasionally, until they are browned, about 8 minutes.

4. Add the mushrooms, salt, thyme, and paprika to the barley and vegetables and cook over medium heat, stirring often, until the mixture is well combined and barley is soft, about more 20 minutes. Spoon into bowls and serve hot.

Per serving: Calories: 235; Fat: 3g; Carbohydrates: 47g; Protein: 7g; Fiber: 10g; Sodium: 618mg

CHICKPEA COCONUT CURRY

GLUTEN-FREE, NUT-FREE, ONE POT, SOY-FREE

PREP TIME: 10 minutes / **COOK TIME:** 25 minutes / **MAKES 4 SERVINGS**

This curry just might become your favorite weekly meal. It goes well with rice or quinoa—I love dividing my bowl into thirds with one part curry, one part grain, and one part greens, like the Sheet-Pan Garlicky Kale (page 148). No matter how you serve it, this dish will never fail to hit the spot.

1 teaspoon extra-virgin olive oil

1 small yellow onion, diced small

3 garlic cloves, minced

1 (2-inch piece) piece fresh ginger, peeled and minced

½ head cauliflower, cut into florets (about 2 cups)

3 teaspoons curry powder

Pinch cayenne pepper

Pinch ground cinnamon

1 teaspoon salt

2 (15-ounce) cans chickpeas, drained and rinsed

1 (15-ounce) can crushed tomatoes

1 (15-ounce) can light unsweetened coconut milk

½ cup frozen peas

2 tablespoons chopped fresh cilantro, for garnish

Black pepper

1. In a large skillet, heat the oil over medium-high heat. Add the onion, garlic, and ginger and cook until fragrant, about 5 minutes.

2. Add the cauliflower and cook until it starts to brown, about 5 minutes. Then add the curry powder, cayenne, cinnamon, salt, chickpeas, tomatoes, and coconut milk and bring to a boil, stirring frequently.

3. Lower the heat to medium-low and simmer until the liquid thickens, about 15 minutes. Add the peas and cook until they are heated through. Spoon the curry into bowls and garnish with cilantro and black pepper.

Per serving: Calories: 335; Fat: 14g; Carbohydrates: 45g; Protein: 14g; Fiber: 10g; Sodium: 892mg

SPICED EGGPLANT AND HUMMUS SANDWICHES

PREP TIME: 10 minutes / **COOK TIME:** 20 minutes / **MAKES 2 SANDWICHES**

Veggie sandwiches have been a staple for me since college, when my crew and I used to make them with smoked Gouda cheese, hummus, avocado, and thick slices of tomatoes. These days I have ditched the cheese and replaced it with smoky roasted eggplant, and its exquisite textures and flavors still thrill me. Cold cuts beware; when the masses find out that sandwiches can be healthy and delicious, you are a goner.

WEEK
4

1 (½-pound) Italian eggplant, cut lengthwise into 4 slices

½ teaspoon salt, plus more for the eggplant

1 tablespoon extra-virgin olive oil

½ teaspoon smoked paprika

½ teaspoon garlic powder

2 red or yellow bell peppers, seeded and halved

4 slices whole-wheat bread

¼ cup store-bought hummus or Garlic Hummus (page 147)

1 cup arugula

1 medium tomato, cut into thick slices

2 tablespoons sesame seeds (optional)

1. Preheat the oven to 425°F.

2. Arrange the eggplant slices on a sheet pan and salt lightly. Let sit for 10 minutes until they release their juices, then rinse the slices and pat dry. Using a sharp knife, score the eggplant slices in a crosshatch pattern. Set aside.

3. In a large bowl, mix together the oil, ½ teaspoon salt, smoked paprika, and garlic powder to make a wet rub. Dredge the eggplant slices in the rub, making sure they are coated well. Arrange them on the sheet pan in a single layer with the crosshatch side up.

CONTINUED ▶

4. Arrange the bell peppers around the eggplant and bake for 10 minutes. Using tongs or a spatula, flip the eggplant and continue to bake for another 10 minutes.

5. When the vegetables are almost done, toast the bread. To assemble the sandwiches, spread the hummus in a thick layer on a slice of toast, add half of the arugula, tomatoes, eggplant, and peppers, sprinkle with sesame seeds (if using), and top with a second slice of toast. Repeat for the second sandwich.

Leftovers Tip: Chop any leftover eggplant into cubes and add it to the Mushroom Barley Soup (page 113) in step 3 or the Marinara Sauce (page 122) in step 1.

Per serving (1 sandwich): **Calories: 357; Fat: 12g; Carbohydrates: 51g; Protein: 13g; Fiber: 12g; Sodium: 959mg**

WHITE BEAN AND KALE LINGUINE

NUT-FREE, ONE POT, QUICK, SOY-FREE

PREP TIME: 10 minutes / **COOK TIME:** 20 minutes / **MAKES 4 SERVINGS**

This filling and comforting 30-minute pasta dinner is a nutritional power-house. The plant-based protein punch from the white beans plus the superfood qualities of kale make it a win-win: feed your body with major fiber and flavor at the same time. This recipe is easy to make yet seems gourmet with the creamy beans, sweet peppers, and savory marinara.

1 pound whole-wheat linguine

2 tablespoons extra-virgin olive oil, divided

½ small yellow onion, diced small

3 garlic cloves, minced

3 sweet baby bell peppers, seeded and diced small

1 (28-ounce) can crushed tomatoes

2 tablespoons tomato paste

½ teaspoon maple syrup

1 cup water

1 (15-ounce) can white cannellini beans, drained and rinsed

Pinch of salt

Pinch of red pepper flakes, plus more for serving (optional)

3 cups stemmed and chopped kale

6 basil leaves, finely chopped

Black pepper

1. Bring a large pot of water to a boil over high heat. Add the pasta and cook according to the package instructions. Drain and set aside.

2. In a large pan, heat the olive oil over medium heat. Add the onion and garlic and sauté until very fragrant, 3 to 5 minutes.

3. Add the bell peppers and cook until the peppers are soft and the onion is browned, about 3 minutes. Add the crushed tomatoes, tomato paste, maple syrup, and water, stir until combined, raise the heat to high, and bring to a boil. Add the beans, salt, and red pepper flakes (if using), stir until combined, and cook for 5 minutes.

CONTINUED ▶

4. Add the kale and stir until just wilted. Add the cooked pasta and toss until evenly coated with the sauce.

5. To serve, spoon into bowls and top the pasta with fresh basil, black pepper, and more red pepper flakes, if desired.

Variation Tip: Try making it with half linguine and half zucchini noodles. The zoodles are so thin and delicate that they will "cook" from the heat of the pasta sauce.

Per serving: Calories: 675; Fat: 10g; Carbohydrates: 131g; Protein: 29g; Fiber: 19g; Sodium: 459mg

PULLED JACKFRUIT TACOS

GLUTEN-FREE, NUT-FREE, QUICK, SOY-FREE

PREP TIME: 5 minutes / **COOK TIME:** 20 minutes / **MAKES 2 SERVINGS**

Jackfruit is a plant-based-eater's dream. The texture and appearance are so similar to shredded pork or chicken, and the flavor is super mild, so it takes on the flavors of whatever sauces or spices you are cooking it with. It's perfect for tacos, sandwiches, or as an addition to soups and stews.

- 1 (15-ounce) can jackfruit, drained and rinsed
- 2 teaspoons extra-virgin olive oil
- ½ small yellow onion, thinly sliced
- ½ green bell pepper, seeded and thinly sliced
- ½ teaspoon salt
- ½ teaspoon chili powder
- ½ teaspoon smoked paprika
- ½ teaspoon garlic powder

- 12 (6-inch) corn tortillas, for serving
- Coleslaw mix or Tangy Cabbage and Kale Slaw (page 144), for serving
- Store-bought salsa or Pico de Gallo (page 172), for serving
- Store-bought guacamole or Super-Simple Guacamole (page 171), for serving (optional)

1. Preheat the oven to 425°F.

2. Shred the jackfruit into small pieces and spread them in an 8-by-8-inch baking dish. Add the olive oil, onion, bell pepper, salt, chili powder, smoked paprika, and garlic powder and gently toss until combined.

3. Bake for 10 minutes. Using a spatula, turn the mixture and continue to bake for another 10 minutes, or until it's slightly crispy.

4. While the mixture is baking, in a large skillet, warm the tortillas over medium-high heat, about 2 minutes on each side. Divide the mixture among the tortillas. Serve topped with coleslaw mix, salsa, and guacamole (if using).

Per serving (3 tacos): Calories: 766; Fat: 17g; Carbohydrates: 140g; Protein: 18g; Fiber: 9g; Sodium: 1,564mg

BBQ TEMPEH SUCCOTASH SKILLET

GLUTEN-FREE, NUT-FREE, QUICK

PREP TIME: 10 minutes / **COOK TIME:** 20 minutes / **MAKES 4 SERVINGS**

The hint of sweet and spicy barbecue sauce tossed into this Southern-influenced stir-fry is heavenly. Collard greens are one of my absolute favorites of the power greens, and they have a great texture and slightly bitter flavor that goes so well with the sweetness of the bell peppers, corn, and sauce.

- 1 (8-ounce) package tempeh, diced
- 2 tablespoons store-bought barbecue sauce or BBQ Sauce (page 181)
- 1 tablespoon extra-virgin olive oil
- 2 garlic cloves, minced
- 1 bunch collard greens, stemmed and chopped
- 1 red bell pepper, seeded and diced
- 1 cup frozen corn
- 2 scallions, white and green parts, thinly sliced
- 2 cups cooked or frozen brown rice
- 1 (15-ounce) can chickpeas, drained and rinsed
- ½ teaspoon salt
- ½ teaspoon black pepper
- ¼ cup water
- 1 avocado, peeled, pitted, quartered, and diced, for serving

1. In a medium bowl, mix together the tempeh and the barbecue sauce until well coated. Set aside.

2. In a large saucepan, heat the olive oil over medium-high heat. Add the garlic and cook until fragrant, 2 to 3 minutes. Add the collard greens and bell pepper and cook, stirring often, until the greens begin to wilt, about 5 minutes.

3. Push the vegetables to one side of the pan. Add the BBQ tempeh and cook for 2 to 3 minutes before stirring it into the vegetables. Add the corn, scallions, rice, chickpeas, salt, pepper, and water and stir until combined. Cover the pan and cook until the vegetables are tender and heated through, 5 to 7 minutes. Spoon into bowls, top with the avocado, and serve.

Per serving: Calories: 448; Fat: 16g; Carbohydrates: 61g; Protein: 20g; Fiber: 11g; Sodium: 518mg

WEEK
4

MEATLESS MEATBALLS WITH QUICK MARINARA SAUCE

PREP TIME: 15 minutes / **COOK TIME:** 30 minutes / **MAKES 4 SERVINGS**

When I was a child, my dad spent hours each weekend making meatballs, and he was immensely proud of his recipe. Big family gatherings almost always had a meatball contest and I learned how to make them at a very young age. It's no different in my home now—these meatless meatballs are revered as a favorite dinner. I replaced the traditional ingredients with a combo of plant-based ones, including oats, nuts, tapioca flour, and flax-seeds. Combining these helps to bind and firm up the balls and give them a great texture and delicious mild flavor.

FOR THE MEATBALLS

1 tablespoon extra-virgin olive oil

½ cup macadamia nuts

1 cup rolled oats

1 (16-ounce) package extra-firm tofu, drained

1 teaspoon tapioca flour

1 tablespoon nutritional yeast

1 teaspoon ground flaxseeds

1 teaspoon onion powder

1 teaspoon garlic powder

1 teaspoon salt

1 teaspoon Italian seasoning

FOR THE QUICK MARINARA

1 teaspoon extra-virgin olive oil

2 garlic cloves, minced

Pinch red pepper flakes

1 (15-ounce) can crushed tomatoes

½ teaspoon maple syrup

¼ teaspoon onion powder

¼ teaspoon Italian seasoning

Salt (optional)

1. **Make the meatballs:** Preheat oven to 400°F. Oil a sheet pan with the olive oil.

2. In a blender or food processor, combine the macadamia nuts and oats and blend until it forms a fine flour. Transfer the mixture to a large bowl.

3. Crumble the tofu with your hands and add it to the bowl. Add the tapioca flour, nutritional yeast, flaxseeds, onion powder, garlic powder, salt, and Italian seasoning and knead together until the mixture is well combined. Form the mixture into 8 balls and arrange them on the prepared sheet pan.

4. Bake for 15 minutes. Using tongs, turn the meatballs and continue to bake for another 15 minutes, or until they are browned and crispy.

5. Make the quick marinara: While the meatballs are baking, in a large saucepan, heat the oil over medium heat. Add the garlic and cook until the garlic is fragrant and slightly golden, 2 to 3 minutes. Add the red pepper flakes, crushed tomatoes, maple syrup, onion powder, and Italian seasoning, stir until combined, and bring to a boil. Lower the heat to medium-low and simmer for 5 minutes. Taste and add salt, if desired.

6. Serve the meatballs topped with the sauce.

> **Leftovers Tip:** The cooked meatballs and the sauce will freeze well, either together or separately, for up to 3 months. To reheat, heat the meatballs in the sauce in a saucepan over medium heat until warmed through.

Per serving (2 meatballs plus ½ cup of the sauce): Calories: 386; Fat: 26g; Carbohydrates: 28g; Protein: 18g; Fiber: 6g; Sodium: 791mg

WEEK
4

RAINBOW SHEPHERD'S PIE

NUT-FREE

PREP TIME: 15 minutes / **COOK TIME:** 45 minutes / **MAKES 4 SERVINGS**

This colorful vegan version of a comfort food classic is the polar opposite of the old standard, in the best way possible. The tempeh and vegetables are coated in a rich, savory gravy and then topped with mashed sweet potatoes. It's plant-based paradise in every bite.

FOR THE TOPPING

- **4 medium sweet potatoes, peeled and diced (about 4 cups)**
- **½ teaspoon salt**
- **1 teaspoon garlic powder**
- **2 tablespoons nutritional yeast**
- **¼ cup unsweetened plant-based milk**

FOR THE FILLING

- **1 (8-ounce) package tempeh**
- **2 teaspoons extra-virgin olive oil**
- **½ small yellow onion, diced small**
- **½ red or yellow bell pepper, diced small**
- **1 large carrot, peeled and diced small**
- **½ cup frozen corn**
- **½ cup frozen peas**
- **2 tablespoons whole-wheat flour**
- **2 tablespoons tomato paste**
- **2 tablespoons low-sodium soy sauce or gluten-free tamari**
- **2 cups water**

1. Preheat the oven to 375°F.

2. **Make the topping:** Put the sweet potatoes in a medium saucepan and cover with enough water to cover completely. Bring to a boil over high heat. Lower the heat to medium and cook until the sweet potatoes are tender, about 15 minutes. Drain and return the potatoes to the saucepan. Add the salt, garlic powder, nutritional yeast, and plant-based milk and, using a potato masher, mash until creamy. Set aside.

3. **Make the filling:** While the potatoes are cooking, in a blender or food processor, pulse the tempeh into very small pieces.

WEEK
4

4. In a large skillet over medium heat, heat the oil. Add the tempeh and onion and cook, stirring often, until the onion and tempeh are lightly browned, about 10 minutes. Add the bell pepper, carrot, corn, and peas and cook until the peppers are fragrant, about 5 minutes.

5. Add the flour and stir until well combined. Add the tomato paste, soy sauce, and water and bring to a boil. Lower the heat to medium and cook, stirring often, until a thick gravy forms.

6. **Assemble the dish:** In an 8-by-8-inch baking dish, spread out the tempeh and veggie mixture. Top with the mashed sweet potatoes, spreading it to the edges. Cover with aluminum foil and bake for 15 minutes, until bubbly.

Per serving: Calories: 322; Fat: 9g; Carbohydrates: 48g; Protein: 17g; Fiber: 7g; Sodium: 668mg

CHICKPEA, BUTTERNUT SQUASH, AND HERB STUFFED PEPPERS

GLUTEN-FREE, NUT-FREE, SOY-FREE

PREP TIME: 5 minutes / **COOK TIME:** 40 minutes / **MAKES 4 SERVINGS**

Stuffed peppers are loved by carnivores and herbivores alike. A hearty flavorful filling of herby rice, chickpeas, and vegetables makes this one a real winner. The perfect weekend afternoon cooking experience, it fills the house with a heavenly aroma of Mediterranean flavors. The lemon and mint really complement the sweet bell peppers and butternut squash.

- 2 teaspoons extra-virgin olive oil
- ½ small yellow onion, diced small
- 3 garlic cloves, minced
- 1 (15-ounce can) chickpeas, drained and rinsed
- 2 cups frozen cubed butternut squash
- 1 teaspoon smoked paprika
- 1 teaspoon maple syrup
- ¼ cup plus 2 tablespoons water, divided
- 1 teaspoon salt
- 1 teaspoon Italian seasoning
- 2 tablespoons chopped fresh parsley
- 2 tablespoons chopped fresh mint
- 2 cups finely chopped baby spinach
- Juice of 1 lemon
- 1 cup frozen or cooked brown rice
- 4 large red or yellow bell peppers

1. In a large skillet, heat the olive oil over medium heat. Add the onion and garlic and cook, stirring often, until fragrant, about 5 minutes. Add the chickpeas, squash, smoked paprika, maple syrup, and ¼ cup of water and cook, stirring constantly, for 5 minutes.

2. Remove from the heat and add the salt, Italian seasoning, parsley, mint, spinach, and lemon juice. Add the brown rice and mix well.

3. Preheat the oven to 400°F.

4. Rinse the bell peppers and pat dry with paper towels. Cut about 2 inches off the top of each pepper. Remove and discard the seeds. Spoon equal amounts of the vegetable-rice mixture into the peppers, packing it in tightly. Cover with the pepper tops.

5. Transfer the stuffed peppers into an 8-by-8-inch baking dish. Pour the remaining 2 tablespoons water into the bottom of the baking dish. Cover the dish with aluminum foil and bake for 30 minutes. Serve hot.

Per serving (1 stuffed pepper): Calories: 254; Fat: 5g; Carbohydrates: 49g; Protein: 9g; Fiber: 8g; Sodium: 724mg

CHOCOLATE PUDDING WITH RASPBERRIES AND MINT

GLUTEN-FREE, NUT-FREE, OIL-FREE

PREP TIME: 20 minutes / **COOK TIME:** 20 minutes / **MAKES 4 SERVINGS**

One of the first things I ever learned to cook as a child was instant pudding. My mom would let me stand up on a chair and stir the pudding as it got thicker and more delicious. This pudding is much different from those little instant boxes—it is higher in protein and made without refined sugars—but even my kids wouldn't know that it isn't junk food.

1 (16-ounce) package silken tofu

1 (15-ounce) can full-fat coconut milk

5 tablespoons unsweetened cocoa powder

6 tablespoons maple syrup

1 tablespoon tapioca flour

1 tablespoon water

16 raspberries, for garnish

4 mint leaves, for garnish

1. In a blender, combine the tofu, coconut milk, cocoa powder, and maple syrup and puree until smooth.

2. Transfer the mixture to a medium saucepan set over medium heat and bring to a gentle boil. Lower the heat to medium.

3. In a small bowl, mix together the tapioca flour and water until smooth to make a slurry. Add the mixture to the saucepan and stir well until combined. Cook for an additional 2 to 3 minutes over medium heat, stirring constantly, to thicken the pudding.

4. Evenly divide the pudding among 4 cups or jars, cover, and refrigerate until chilled. The pudding will get firmer as it cools.

5. To serve, garnish each portion with 4 raspberries and 1 mint leaf. The pudding will last up to 4 days, covered, in the refrigerator.

Per serving: Calories: 480; Fat: 29g; Carbohydrates: 29g; Protein: 15g; Fiber: 9g; Sodium: 28mg

CHAPTER EIGHT

MORE RECIPES FOR PLANT-BASED LIVING

Peanut Butter Cookies,
page 169

BAKED FLAXSEED-BATTERED FRENCH TOAST

PREP TIME: 10 minutes / **COOK TIME:** 15 minutes / **MAKES 4 SERVINGS**

In this easy recipe the ground flaxseeds do a wonderful job mimicking the silky texture of eggs. My picky kids love the hints of vanilla and cinnamon, and I love that they are getting extra fiber, protein, and omega-3 fatty acids in every bite!

¼ cup ground flaxseeds

1½ cups unsweetened
  plant-based milk, divided

Olive oil cooking spray

1 tablespoon ground cinnamon

1 teaspoon vanilla extract

3 tablespoons maple syrup,
  plus more for serving

8 slices whole-grain bread

1. In a medium bowl, combine the flaxseeds and ½ cup of plant-based milk. Let the mixture stand for 10 minutes to give the flaxseeds time to absorb the liquid and thicken, which will give them an eggy consistency.

2. Preheat the oven to 400°F. Spray a sheet pan with olive oil cooking spray.

3. Add the remaining 1 cup plant-based milk, the cinnamon, vanilla, and maple syrup to the flax mixture and mix until combined. Dip each slice of bread into the flax mixture, making sure to completely cover in the liquid. Let any excess drip back into the bowl and then put the slices on the sheet pan.

4. Bake for 10 minutes. Using a spatula, carefully flip the bread and bake for 5 minutes. Serve with maple syrup.

Leftovers Tip: Wrap leftovers tightly in plastic wrap and refrigerate for up to 3 days. To reheat, bake at 400°F for 5 minutes.

Per serving (2 slices): Calories: 272; Fat: 7g; Carbohydrates: 42g; Protein: 11g; Fiber: 7g; Sodium: 249mg

GLUTEN-FREE BLUEBERRY BLENDER PANCAKES

GLUTEN-FREE, NUT-FREE, QUICK

PREP TIME: 5 minutes / **COOK TIME:** 10 minutes / **MAKES 2 SERVINGS**

This recipe can be thrown together in a jiffy on a busy weekday morning, or you can prepare the batter the night before and have it ready to quickly cook the pancakes the next day.

1 cup unsweetened
  plant-based milk

1 teaspoon apple cider vinegar

1 tablespoon extra-virgin olive oil

3 tablespoons maple syrup, plus
  more for serving

1 teaspoon vanilla extract

1 tablespoon baking powder

1 cup gluten-free flour

½ teaspoon salt

1 tablespoon coconut oil

½ cup fresh or frozen blueberries

1. In a blender, combine the plant-based milk and apple cider vinegar and let sit for 3 minutes to make a faux buttermilk.

2. Add the olive oil, maple syrup, and vanilla to the "buttermilk" and blend until very smooth.

3. Add the baking powder, flour, and salt and pulse until just combined. Do not blend long.

4. In a griddle or a large skillet, melt the coconut oil over medium heat. When the griddle is hot, pour the pancake batter on the griddle to make 3-inch pancakes, leaving about 1 inch between them. Drop blueberries onto each pancake as they are cooking. Cook until the pancakes have bubbles in the middle, 3 to 5 minutes. Using a spatula, flip the pancakes and continue to cook until browned, another 3 to 5 minutes. Serve with maple syrup.

Per serving (4 pancakes): Calories: 565; Fat: 20g; Carbohydrates: 87g; Protein: 16g; Fiber: 9g; Sodium: 718mg

SUPERSEED AND NUT BREAKFAST COOKIES

QUICK, SOY-FREE

PREP TIME: 10 minutes / **COOK TIME:** 15 minutes / **MAKES 12 COOKIES**

Breakfast cookies are a game changer on a busy morning, and these have the power and nutrition of a bar in a quick handheld meal. They are perfect for the car ride to work or to munch while you get ready for your day. Disguised as dessert, these grab-and-go cookies are a great source of protein and fats that will give you the needed fuel to start your day deliciously.

1 tablespoon ground flaxseeds

3 tablespoons water

1 cup whole-wheat flour

1 cup rolled oats

2 tablespoons hemp hearts

2 tablespoons pumpkin seeds

2 tablespoons sunflower seeds

3 tablespoons raisins

1 tablespoon baking powder

1 teaspoon salt

1 tablespoon ground cinnamon

2 tablespoons chopped walnuts

3 tablespoons coconut oil, melted

**2 tablespoons natural
  peanut butter**

½ cup maple syrup

1. Preheat the oven to 350°F. Line a sheet pan with parchment paper.

2. In a small bowl, mix together the flaxseeds and water to form a "flax egg." Set aside.

3. In a large bowl, mix together the flour, oats, hemp hearts, pumpkin seeds, sunflower seeds, raisins, baking powder, salt, cinnamon, and walnuts.

4. Add the coconut oil, flax egg, peanut butter, and maple syrup to the flour mixture and stir well until combined.

5. Using a spoon, scoop 2 tablespoons of batter per cookie onto the prepared sheet pan, leaving at least 1 inch between them. Bake for 10 to 12 minutes, or until the cookies are firm and golden brown.

Per serving (2 cookies): Calories: 351; Fat: 16g; Carbohydrates: 49g; Protein: 8g; Fiber: 6g; Sodium: 402mg

STUFFED BREAKFAST SWEET POTATOES

PREP TIME: 5 minutes / **COOK TIME:** 10 minutes / **MAKES 2 SERVINGS**

I discovered this delicious combo a few years ago. Who would have known that a baked sweet potato would pair so well with these toppings? I love this breakfast because it is delicious, satisfying, and is ready in no time at all.

2 medium sweet potatoes

2 tablespoons almond butter

2 tablespoons plain plant-based yogurt

2 tablespoons maple syrup

½ cup store-bought granola or Crispy, Crunchy Granola (page 184)

1. Scrub the sweet potatoes well. Using a fork, poke holes all over each potato.

2. Put the potatoes on a microwave-safe plate and microwave on high for 2-minute intervals, turning them over after each, until the sweet potatoes are easily pierced with a fork. Alternately, you can bake them in the oven on a sheet pan at 400°F for about 40 minutes, until it can be easily pierced with a fork.

3. Let the sweet potatoes cool for a few minutes, just until you can handle them. Cut each potato lengthwise down the middle and expose the insides. Using a fork, lightly mash the insides and open the potato wider. Drizzle each with almond butter, yogurt, and maple syrup and sprinkle the granola on top. Serve hot.

Variation Tip: To make a savory breakfast sweet potato, dollop with Plant-Based Queso Dip (page 139) and cooked chopped broccoli florets, or top with plain plant-based yogurt and chopped scallions.

Per serving: Calories: 410; Fat: 16g; Carbohydrates: 62g; Protein: 9g; Fiber: 8g; Sodium: 160mg

PLANT-BASED MANGO LASSI SMOOTHIES

5 INGREDIENTS, GLUTEN-FREE, NO COOK, NUT-FREE, QUICK

PREP TIME: 5 minutes / **MAKES 2 SERVINGS**

A lassi is a sweet yogurt-based drink that originated in India. When I was an omnivore, I could never pass up a heavenly lassi when visiting an Indian restaurant. I was inspired to create this plant-based version with exquisitely delicious mangoes combined with plant-based yogurt, bananas, and flax. This makes an awesome-tasting smoothie. Enjoy this treat year-round by storing frozen mangos in your freezer. This smoothie is excellent for digestion and wonderful on its own or as an accompaniment to a spicy curry meal for its cooling properties.

2 frozen sliced bananas

2 cups frozen mango chunks

2 cups unsweetened plant-based milk

1 cup plain plant-based yogurt

2 tablespoons ground flaxseeds

In a blender, combine the bananas, mango, plant-based milk, plant-based yogurt, and flaxseeds and puree until smooth. Pour into 2 glasses and enjoy immediately.

Per serving: Calories: 391; Fat: 8g; Carbohydrates: 71g; Protein: 16g; Fiber: 8g; Sodium: 207mg

LOADED SWEET APPLE "NACHOS"

PREP TIME: 5 minutes / **MAKES 2 SERVINGS**

These sweet "nachos" are the stuff dreams are made of. While this recipe has nothing to do with cheesy corn chips, it will have you licking your fingers and dipping like crazy! This is a great snack for two to share, though it's easy to scale up or down based on your needs.

3 apples, any kind, cored and cut into thin wedges

1 teaspoon ground cinnamon

2 tablespoons almond butter or tahini

2 tablespoons plain plant-based yogurt

1 tablespoon maple syrup

1 tablespoon raisins

2 tablespoons chopped nuts of choice

2 tablespoons unsweetened coconut flakes

1 tablespoon cacao nibs or vegan refined-sugar-free chocolate chips (optional)

On a large plate, spread out the apple wedges in a single layer and sprinkle with the cinnamon. Drizzle the apples with the almond butter, yogurt, and maple syrup. Sprinkle the raisins, nuts, coconut, and cacao nibs (if using) over the top.

Ingredient Tip: Cacao nibs are crumbled cacao beans, which is the same bean used to make chocolate. In this form they are suitable for a whole-food, plant-based diet because they are free of dairy and refined sugar. Available in most health-food stores, they are a nice topper for smoothie bowls, yogurt parfaits, and other sweet treats.

Variation Tip: Make it a watermelon "pizza" instead by cutting a 1-inch-thick slice of watermelon, slicing it into wedges, and layering the same toppings on each piece.

Per serving: Calories: 361; Fat: 15g; Carbohydrates: 58g; Protein: 7g; Fiber: 10g; Sodium: 18mg

ZINGY MELON AND MANGO SALAD

5 INGREDIENTS, GLUTEN-FREE, NO COOK, NUT-FREE,
OIL-FREE, ONE BOWL, QUICK, SOY-FREE

PREP TIME: 5 minutes / **MAKES 2 SERVINGS**

I love the juxtaposition of sweet and savory in this salad. The mango and melon flavors pop in a really special way with the addition of lime, chili powder, and fresh cilantro. Depending on the size of your fruit chunks, this can be eaten as is or, if chopped small, used like a salsa on tacos or with chips.

1 large mango, peeled, pitted, and cut into 1-inch pieces (about 1 cup)

½ small cantaloupe or watermelon, peeled and cut into 1-inch pieces (about 2 cups)

Juice of 1 lime

¼ cup chopped fresh cilantro

1 teaspoon chili powder

In a large bowl, combine the mango and cantaloupe. Add the lime juice and cilantro and gently toss until combined. To serve, spoon into bowls and sprinkle with chili powder.

Ingredient Tip: Mangoes can be tricky to cut. Always cut ½ inch off one end first to have a flat surface to balance the mango on your cutting board. Cut the "meat" off the mango before peeling the skin to avoid cutting your fingers—mangos are slippery.

Variation Tip: Add a diced avocado and ½ cup macadamia nuts to make a heartier salad that can be served over some crunchy romaine lettuce for a light weekday lunch.

Per serving: Calories: 171; Fat: 1g; Carbohydrates: 42g; Protein: 3g; Fiber: 5g; Sodium: 70mg

PLANT-BASED QUESO DIP

GLUTEN-FREE, OIL-FREE, QUICK

PREP TIME: 5 minutes / **COOK TIME:** 20 minutes / **MAKES 3 CUPS**

This deliciously "cheesy" plant-based queso is tasty with tortilla chips, drizzled on tacos, or even as a dip for roasted vegetables.

1 cup raw cashews

1 cup cubed butternut squash

1 yellow or orange bell pepper, seeded and cut into quarters

2 cups plus 1 teaspoon water, divided

1 cup unsweetened plant-based milk

1 tablespoon nutritional yeast

½ teaspoon salt

½ teaspoon onion powder

½ teaspoon garlic powder

¼ teaspoon smoked paprika

½ jalapeño pepper, seeded and minced (optional)

1 teaspoon tapioca flour

1. In a medium saucepan, combine the cashews, butternut squash, bell pepper, and 2 cups of water and bring to a boil. Lower the heat to medium and cook until the squash and cashews are soft, about 15 minutes. Drain and transfer the ingredients to a blender or food processor.

2. Add the plant-based milk, nutritional yeast, salt, onion powder, garlic powder, and smoked paprika and blend until smooth and creamy.

3. Transfer the mixture back to the saucepan and slowly bring to a boil over medium-high heat, stirring often. Add the jalapeño (if desired) and cook for 2 to 3 minutes.

4. In a small bowl, mix together the tapioca flour and the remaining 1 teaspoon water to make a slurry. Add the slurry to the cheese sauce and cook, stirring constantly, until the sauce is thick and creamy, about 2 more minutes. Refrigerate leftovers for up to 4 days.

Per serving (¼ cup): Calories: 85; Fat: 6g; Carbohydrates: 7g; Protein: 3g; Fiber: 1g; Sodium: 109mg

SWEET POTATO FRIES WITH MAPLE, MINT, AND TAHINI DIPPING SAUCE

GLUTEN-FREE, NUT-FREE, SOY-FREE

PREP TIME: 5 minutes / **COOK TIME:** 30 minutes / **MAKES 2 SERVINGS**

Everyone loves fries, but this healthier twist on the traditional is a show-stopper. Crispy, savory, and sweet, these potato wedges are the perfect side dish for Brown Rice and Black Bean Veggie Burgers (page 34) and Tempeh and Lentil Sloppy Joes (page 65), or as a simple and satisfying snack! You can serve them with any sauce you like, such as Sugar-Free Ketchup (page 180), Super-Simple Guacamole (page 171), or Lemon Aioli (page 142), but I think the sauce here complements the flavors perfectly.

FOR THE FRIES

3 sweet potatoes, cut into wedges

2 teaspoons extra-virgin olive oil

½ teaspoon salt

½ teaspoon garlic powder

FOR THE SAUCE

⅓ cup tahini

1 tablespoon maple syrup

½ teaspoon salt

Juice of 1 lemon

4 mint leaves

1 garlic clove

Pinch red pepper flakes (optional)

1. Preheat the oven to 400°F.

2. **Make the fries:** In a large bowl, combine the potatoes, olive oil, salt, and garlic powder and toss until the potatoes are well coated with the seasonings.

3. Spread out the sweet potatoes in a single layer on a sheet pan and bake for 15 minutes. Using a spatula, turn the potatoes, then continue to bake for another 15 minutes.

4. Make the sauce: While the fries are in the oven, in a blender, combine the tahini, maple syrup, salt, lemon juice, mint, and garlic and blend until smooth. Transfer to a small bowl, add the red pepper flakes (if using), and stir well. Cover and refrigerate until ready to use.

Per serving: Calories: 479; Fat: 26g; Carbohydrates: 57g; Protein: 10g; Fiber: 10g; Sodium: 2,481mg

HERBED SMASHED POTATOES WITH LEMON AIOLI

GLUTEN-FREE, NUT-FREE

PREP TIME: 5 minutes / **COOK TIME:** 1 hour / **MAKES 4 SERVINGS**

These smashed potatoes are a snacker's dream and the perfect side dish to go with the Portobello Mushroom Burgers with Arugula Pesto (page 94) or Spiced Eggplant and Hummus Sandwiches (page 115). Garlicky and super savory, they are lifted to a new level by the lemony aioli. This method of cooking produces the tastiest potatoes you have ever eaten, with the extra surface area and exposed potato from the smashing turning a gorgeous golden color and forming an exquisite crispiness.

FOR THE POTATOES

12 small red potatoes

2 tablespoons extra-virgin olive oil

1 teaspoon garlic powder

½ teaspoon salt

1 teaspoon Italian seasoning

2 tablespoons finely chopped fresh parsley

FOR THE LEMON AIOLI

½ cup store-bought plant-based mayonnaise or Plant-Based Mayo (page 178)

Juice of 1 lemon

1 garlic clove, minced

1. Preheat the oven to 400°F.

2. **Make the potatoes:** Put the potatoes in a large pot over high heat, add enough water to cover, and bring to a boil. Cook for 15 minutes. Drain well and pat the potatoes dry with a clean kitchen towel. Transfer the potatoes to a large bowl.

3. Add the olive oil, garlic powder, and salt and gently toss until all the potatoes are coated in the seasonings. Spread out the seasoned potatoes in one layer on a sheet pan.

4. Bake for 15 minutes. Using tongs, turn the potatoes and continue to bake for another 15 minutes. Using the back of a fork, smash the potatoes flat. Sprinkle them with the Italian seasoning and bake for an additional 10 minutes, or until crispy and golden.

5. Make the lemon aioli: While the potatoes finish baking, in a small bowl, mix together the mayo, lemon juice, and garlic.

6. Transfer the potatoes to a platter, sprinkle with parsley, and serve with the lemon aioli on the side for dipping.

Variation Tip: For an amazing chilled potato salad, combine the aioli with any left-over potatoes.

Per serving: Calories: 520; Fat: 17g; Carbohydrates: 84g; Protein: 12g; Fiber: 9g; Sodium: 616mg

TANGY CABBAGE AND KALE SLAW

5 INGREDIENTS, GLUTEN-FREE, NO COOK, NUT-FREE,
ONE BOWL, QUICK, SOY-FREE

PREP TIME: 10 minutes / **MAKES 3 CUPS**

Because I am a huge fan of cabbage, I have always loved coleslaw. I prefer the vinegary variety to the creamy mayonnaise version, so that's what I've channeled here. This slaw is super simple and is best on tacos or in sandwiches where it complements the other ingredients. It is crunchy, fresh, and super zesty. Bonus is that it can come together in 10 minutes or less.

8 ounces shredded cabbage

½ bunch fresh cilantro, chopped

1 scallion, white and green parts, chopped

½ bunch kale, stemmed (if desired) and chopped small

½ teaspoon salt

1 teaspoon extra-virgin olive oil

Juice of 2 limes

In a large bowl, combine the cabbage, cilantro, scallion, kale, salt, olive oil, and lime juice and mix well with your hands. Store in an airtight container for up to 3 days in the refrigerator.

Ingredient Tip: For extra convenience, buy a 16-ounce bag of precut cabbage-and-carrot slaw and use that instead of the cabbage and kale combo.

Per serving (¾ cup): Calories: 43; Fat: 1g; Carbohydrates: 8g; Protein: 2g; Fiber: 2g; Sodium: 314mg

OVEN-ROASTED DIJON VEGGIES

5 INGREDIENTS, GLUTEN-FREE, NUT-FREE, QUICK, SOY-FREE

PREP TIME: 5 minutes / **COOK TIME:** 20 minutes / **MAKES 4 SERVINGS**

There is nothing I love more than perfectly roasted vegetables. The way a hot oven caramelizes the sugars really enhances their flavors. The key is to cut starchy vegetables like potatoes and squashes smaller so that they cook faster, and vegetables with high water content like broccoli and zucchini larger so they will cook slower to make sure that they're all finished at the same time.

½ **large head cauliflower, cut into florets (about 2 cups)**

½ **large head broccoli, cut into florets (about 2 cups)**

1 **red or yellow bell pepper, seeded and cut into 2-inch-thick slices**

2 **carrots, peeled and cut into 1-inch rounds**

1 **teaspoon extra-virgin olive oil**

1 **teaspoon Dijon mustard**

½ **teaspoon salt**

1. Preheat oven to 425°F.

2. In a large bowl, combine the cauliflower, broccoli, bell pepper, carrots, olive oil, Dijon mustard, and salt and toss until the veggies are well coated with seasonings.

3. Transfer the vegetables to a sheet pan and bake for 10 minutes. Using a spatula, turn the veggies and continue to bake for another 10 minutes, or until they are browned and slightly crispy outside and tender inside. Oven temperatures vary, so if your veggies are not done yet, continue to bake in increments of 5 minutes until cooked to your desired doneness.

Variation Tip: Instead of broccoli, use an 8-ounce package of white mushrooms.

Per serving: Calories: 64; Fat: 1g; Carbohydrates: 13g; Protein: 3g; Fiber: 4g; Sodium: 376mg

CRISPY BAKED CHICKPEAS

5 INGREDIENTS, GLUTEN-FREE, NUT-FREE, QUICK, SOY-FREE

PREP TIME: 5 minutes / **COOK TIME:** 25 minutes / **MAKES 1½ CUPS**

Crispy chickpeas are one of my favorite snacks, and I make a batch of these at least once a week. They add crunchiness and body to a light meal, and they also pack in the protein and fiber, which is a win-win. Since these chickpeas are oven-baked and not deep-fried, they get crispy on the outside but are still meaty and creamy on the inside. They are a great addition to Butternut Squash and White Bean Mac and Cheeze (page 42) or Avocado Toast with Tomato and Hemp Hearts (page 109).

1 (15-ounce) can chickpeas, drained and rinsed

1 tablespoon extra-virgin olive oil

½ teaspoon smoked paprika

½ teaspoon salt

¼ teaspoon garlic powder

1. Preheat the oven to 425°F.

2. In a medium bowl, combine the chickpeas, olive oil, smoked paprika, salt, and garlic powder and toss until combined. Spread out the seasoned chickpeas on a sheet pan and bake for 15 minutes. Using a spatula, turn the chickpeas and continue to bake for another 10 minutes, or until crispy.

Leftovers Tip: Refrigerate in an airtight container for up to 5 days. To reheat, spread out the chickpeas in a single layer on a baking sheet and bake at 400°F oven for 5 minutes to re-crisp them.

Variation Tip: Instead of smoked paprika and garlic, toss the chickpeas with 2 teaspoons of spicy Cajun seasoning or 2 teaspoons of za'atar and bake as instructed. You can also toss them in ½ teaspoon of powdered wasabi after baking for added heat.

Per serving (1 cup): Calories: 147; Fat: 6g; Carbohydrates: 18g; Protein: 5g; Fiber: 5g; Sodium: 546mg

GARLIC HUMMUS

GLUTEN-FREE, NO COOK, NUT-FREE, QUICK, SOY-FREE

PREP TIME: 10 minutes / **MAKES 3 CUPS**

I first discovered hummus in college back in the early '90s. It took me a few years to realize that making it at home was almost as easy as cutting up the carrot sticks for dipping. Nowadays, making homemade hummus is second nature, and the variations are endless. This version is my classic—a little spicy from the garlic, and super lemony and creamy. It goes great with crunchy raw veggies or chips, spread on a sandwich, or thinned out with a bit of water and used as a salad dressing. For this reason, I always jokingly refer to it as "yummus."

3 garlic cloves

2 (15-ounce) cans chickpeas, drained and rinsed

3 tablespoons extra-virgin olive oil, plus more as needed

Juice of 2 lemons

¼ cup tahini

½ teaspoon salt

½ teaspoon ground cumin

1 tablespoon sesame seeds, for garnish (optional)

In a blender, combine the garlic, chickpeas, olive oil, lemon juice, tahini, salt, and cumin and blend until smooth and creamy. Add a bit more oil or water if you prefer a thinner consistency. To serve, spoon it into a bowl, drizzle with a little more olive oil, and garnish with sesame seeds (if using).

Variation Tip: For color and a slight flavor variation, add a roasted red pepper or a peeled and boiled beet to the blender. You can also add 1 tablespoon of ground turmeric for a superfood immunity boost! If you like spicy foods, add a jalapeño and a handful of fresh cilantro to the other ingredients and blend.

Per serving (2 tablespoons): Calories: 58; Fat: 4g; Carbohydrates: 5g; Protein: 2g; Fiber: 2g; Sodium: 92mg

SHEET-PAN GARLICKY KALE

5 INGREDIENTS, GLUTEN-FREE, NUT-FREE, ONE PAN, QUICK, SOY-FREE

PREP TIME: 5 minutes / **COOK TIME:** 15 minutes / **MAKES 2 SERVINGS**

Fun fact: I actually have only two working burners in my kitchen, so I discovered this method of cooking greens out of necessity. Little did I know when I first tried it that this would turn out to be one of my favorite ways to prepare them! Even better, there's no need to dry your greens well after washing—the greens actually cook better if the leaves retain some water from their bath—it will prevent the kale from turning crispy.

---

2 garlic cloves, minced

2 teaspoons extra-virgin olive oil

1 bunch kale, roughly chopped

¼ teaspoon salt

¼ teaspoon black pepper

¼ teaspoon garlic powder

1. Preheat the oven to 400°F.

2. In a large bowl, combine the garlic, olive oil, kale, salt, black pepper, and garlic powder and toss until well combined. Spread out the kale on a sheet pan and bake for 10 minutes. Using a spatula, turn the kale and continue to cook for another 5 minutes, until the kale is wilted and bright green.

Cooking Tip: I like to eat the stems on greens like kale and collards, but if you are new to the green life, it's perfectly fine to remove the thick stems if they seem unappetizing to you.

Variation Tip: This recipe works very well with all greens. Shorten the cooking time by 5 minutes for more tender greens like spinach, chard, dandelion greens, or mustard greens. Add 5 minutes for broccoli rabe (or rapini).

Per serving: Calories: 144; Fat: 6g; Carbohydrates: 19g; Protein: 9g; Fiber: 7g; Sodium: 368mg

BLACK BEAN TORTAS

NUT-FREE, ONE PAN, QUICK

PREP TIME: 5 minutes / **COOK TIME:** 15 minutes / **MAKES 4 SANDWICHES**

The first time I saw a Mexican torta I was intrigued. Beans on a sandwich? But once I tried one, I was captivated by the delicious and fresh flavors. Traditionally a torta is a giant Mexican sandwich filled with beans, meat, and cheese. This one is inspired by the original, but it's made entirely plant-based. My house is full of bean lovers, so we have these all the time. Make sure to have a napkin handy—they're messy, but the unforgettable flavors make it worth it.

1 (15-ounce) can black beans, drained and rinsed

½ teaspoon onion powder

½ teaspoon garlic powder

¼ teaspoon salt

¼ cup water

4 teaspoons store-bought mayonnaise or Plant-Based Mayo (page 178)

4 whole-wheat bulkie rolls or burger buns, sliced in half crosswise

1 avocado, peeled, pitted, cut into quarters, and sliced, for serving

¼ cup store-bought salsa or Pico de Gallo (page 172)

2 cups shredded lettuce

¼ cup chopped fresh cilantro

1. In a medium saucepan, combine the black beans, onion powder, garlic powder, salt, and water and bring to a boil. Turn off the heat. Using a potato masher, break up the beans and mash them until they resemble a thick black paste.

2. Spread mayo on the cut sides of the bulkie rolls. In a large skillet over medium heat, toast the bulkie rolls, cut-sides down, until golden, about 3 minutes.

3. To assemble the torta, layer the beans, sliced avocado, salsa, lettuce, and cilantro on one half of the rolls, top with the other half, and serve immediately.

Per serving (1 sandwich): Calories: 312; Fat: 11g; Carbohydrates: 46g; Protein: 11g; Fiber: 13g; Sodium: 543mg

QUICK AND EASY FALAFEL PITAS

PREP TIME: 5 minutes / **COOK TIME:** 20 minutes / **MAKES 4 WRAPS**

I love falafel. The crispy and flavorful Middle Eastern specialty has always captivated me. Mine are less labor intensive, a bit softer textured, and much lighter on the oil than traditional falafels. Try them in a wrap or on a salad. I find that rolling the pita around the fillings is less messy, but you can also cut the pitas in half and stuff them. I recommend drizzling these with the dipping sauce from the Sweet Potato Fries (page 140) or with Garlic Hummus (page 147).

Olive oil cooking spray

1 (15-ounce) can chickpeas, drained and rinsed

1 garlic clove, minced

2 tablespoons minced fresh parsley, or 2 teaspoons dried parsley

½ teaspoon salt

½ teaspoon ground cumin

3 tablespoons whole-wheat flour

½ teaspoon baking soda

4 (6-inch) whole-wheat pita breads

8 tablespoons store-bought hummus or Garlic Hummus (page 147)

3 ounces spring mix or arugula (3 to 4 cups)

2 tomatoes, cut into slices

1. Preheat the oven to 400°F. Spray a sheet pan with cooking spray.

2. In a large bowl, mash the chickpeas with a fork or potato masher. Add the garlic, parsley, salt, cumin, flour, and baking soda and mix well to form a crumbly and sticky mixture.

3. Using your hands, form the mixture into 8 balls, using about 2 tablespoons for each one, and put them on the prepared baking sheet. Bake for 10 minutes. Using tongs, carefully turn the balls and continue to bake for another 10 minutes.

4. To warm the pita breads, place them directly on a rack in the oven and bake for 2 minutes, until they are more pliable.

5. To assemble, spread 2 tablespoons of hummus in the middle of each pita and top with spring mix, sliced tomatoes, and 2 falafel balls. Fold the pita around the fillings.

Variation Tip: Make the falafel balls into 4 patties instead to make falafel burgers. Cook for 20 minutes in a 400°F oven, turning them once halfway through the baking time.

Per serving (1 wrap): Calories: 341; Fat: 6g; Carbohydrates: 62g; Protein: 14g; Fiber: 11g; Sodium: 936mg

BBQ JACKFRUIT SANDWICHES

NUT-FREE, ONE PAN, SOY-FREE

PREP TIME: 5 minutes / **COOK TIME:** 30 minutes / **MAKES 2 SERVINGS**

Jackfruit is the perfect vehicle for barbecue sauce. This filling is great on its own or paired with some crunchy cabbage slaw and your favorite sandwich toppings. The result is decadent and delicious, and I can't wait to wow you with this recipe.

---

1 (15-ounce) can jackfruit, drained and shredded
2 teaspoons extra-virgin olive oil
½ medium yellow onion, finely chopped
2 garlic cloves, finely chopped
2 teaspoons maple syrup
1 tablespoon molasses
1 teaspoon apple cider vinegar

3 tablespoons tomato paste
1 teaspoon smoked paprika
½ teaspoon salt
½ cup water
2 whole-wheat burger buns
1 cup store-bought coleslaw or Tangy Cabbage and Kale Slaw (page 144)

1. Preheat the oven to 400°F.

2. In an 8-by-8-inch baking dish, combine the jackfruit, olive oil, onion, and garlic and bake for 10 minutes. Using a spatula, turn the jackfruit and continue to bake for 10 more minutes.

3. In a small bowl, mix together the maple syrup, molasses, apple cider vinegar, tomato paste, smoked paprika, salt, and water. Add the sauce to the jackfruit, mix well, and bake for 10 more minutes

4. To serve, pile the barbecue jackfruit on the buns and top with the slaw.

Per serving (1 sandwich): Calories: 430; Fat: 8g; Carbohydrates: 88g; Protein: 10g; Fiber: 7g; Sodium: 828mg

GREEN POWER RICE BOWLS

GLUTEN-FREE, NUT-FREE, QUICK

PREP TIME: 10 minutes / **COOK TIME:** 15 minutes / **MAKES 2 BOWLS**

This recipe is perfectly balanced with protein from the peas and hemp seeds, healthy fats from the avocado, nutrients from all the wonderful greens, and a nice slow, steady burn from the brown rice.

---

1 bunch kale, roughly chopped

1 teaspoon extra-virgin olive oil

½ teaspoon garlic powder

¼ teaspoon salt

1 cup frozen peas

1 cup fresh or frozen broccoli florets

¼ cup hemp hearts

1 Persian cucumber, thinly sliced

1 teaspoon sesame oil

1 teaspoon low-sodium soy sauce or gluten-free tamari

1 teaspoon rice vinegar

1 teaspoon maple syrup

1 cup cooked brown rice

1 avocado, peeled, pitted, and sliced

1. Preheat the oven to 425°F.

2. In a large bowl, combine the kale, olive oil, garlic powder, salt, peas, and broccoli and toss until well combined. Spread out the mixture on a sheet pan and bake for 15 minutes. Check the oven every 5 minutes and turn the mixture so that the kale only gets slightly crispy.

3. Add the hemp hearts to the cooked vegetables and toss until well combined. Set aside.

4. In a small bowl, mix together the cucumber, sesame oil, soy sauce, rice vinegar, and maple syrup.

5. To assemble the bowls, arrange the ingredients in sections: rice; kale, broccoli, and pea mixture; cucumbers; and avocado. Drizzle the remaining dressing from the cucumbers over the bowls and serve.

Per serving (1 bowl): Calories: 604; Fat: 32g; Carbohydrates: 67g; Protein: 24g; Fiber: 21g; Sodium: 468mg

BEET SUSHI AND AVOCADO POKE BOWLS

NUT-FREE

PREP TIME: 20 minutes / **COOK TIME:** 20 minutes / **MAKES 2 SERVINGS**

Sushi has always been a favorite of mine, and when I realized that plant-based sushi was just as delicious as the real thing, I was overjoyed. You'll be shocked it is not tuna! Red beets look just like maguro, and golden or pink beets look a lot like salmon. The dressing really kicks up the flavors, but if you don't like spicy food, just omit the wasabi. Gluten-free tamari or coconut aminos can be used in place of the soy sauce for a gluten-free dish that's lower in sodium.

- 2 red beets (about 3 ounces each), trimmed and peeled
- 3 cups water
- 2 teaspoons low-sodium soy sauce or gluten-free tamari
- ½ teaspoon wasabi paste (optional)
- 1 tablespoon maple syrup
- 1 teaspoon sesame oil
- 1 teaspoon rice vinegar
- 1 cup frozen shelled edamame
- 1 cup cooked brown rice
- 1 cucumber, peeled and cut into matchsticks
- 2 carrots, cut into matchsticks
- 1 avocado, peeled, pitted, and sliced
- 1 scallion, green and white parts, chopped small, for garnish
- 2 tablespoons sesame seeds, for garnish (optional)

1. In a medium saucepan, combine the beets and water and bring to a boil over high heat. Lower the heat to medium and cook until they are tender but not mushy, about 15 minutes. Drain, rinse, and set aside to cool.

2. In a small bowl, make the dressing by mixing together the soy sauce, wasabi (if using), maple syrup, sesame oil, and rice vinegar and set aside.

3. When the beets are cooled, slide off the skins. Using a sharp knife, cut the beets into very thin slices to resemble tuna sashimi. Put the beet slices in a small bowl and top with 1 teaspoon of the dressing. Set aside to marinate.

4. Put the edamame in a microwave-safe bowl, add water to cover, and cook in the microwave for 1 minute. Drain and set aside.

5. To assemble the bowls, divide the rice between 2 bowls. Top each bowl with the sliced beets, rice, cucumbers, carrots, edamame, and avocado and drizzle with the remaining dressing. Garnish with the scallions and sesame seeds (if using).

Variation Tip: Make smoked "salmon" instead, using carrots! Peel 2 large carrots and cut them in half. Boil in water for about 5 minutes, until slightly soft. Cut as thin as you can. In a bowl, mix together ½ teaspoon smoked paprika, ½ teaspoon maple syrup, and 1 teaspoon low-sodium soy sauce or gluten-free tamari. Add the carrots and let marinate. Add to the bowls along with the other ingredients.

Per serving: Calories: 488; Fat: 22g; Carbohydrates: 63g; Protein: 16g; Fiber: 18g; Sodium: 285mg

SESAME SOBA NOODLE SALAD

GLUTEN-FREE, NUT-FREE, QUICK

PREP TIME: 10 minutes / **COOK TIME:** 10 minutes / **MAKES 4 SERVINGS**

I could happily eat my weight in noodles. If you aren't familiar, soba noodles are Japanese buckwheat noodles, available in most Asian sections at the supermarket. If you cannot find them, rice noodles or even whole-wheat spaghetti are acceptable substitutes and fine vehicles for the tasty dressing!

8 ounces gluten-free buckwheat soba noodles

2 teaspoons sesame oil, divided

3 teaspoons rice vinegar

2 teaspoons maple syrup

1 teaspoon low-sodium soy sauce or gluten-free tamari

4 cups mixed green lettuces

2 cucumbers, sliced

2 cups shredded red cabbage

2 carrots, grated or thinly sliced

¼ cup sesame seeds

1 avocado, peeled, pitted, cut into quarters, and sliced

¼ teaspoon red pepper flakes (optional)

1. Bring a pot of water to a boil over high heat. Add the soba noodles and cook according to the package instructions. Drain and toss with 1 teaspoon of sesame oil.

2. In a small bowl, mix together the rice vinegar, maple syrup, soy sauce, and the remaining 1 teaspoon sesame oil. Set aside.

3. To assemble the salad, layer the mixed greens, sliced cucumbers, shredded cabbage, and carrots in 4 bowls and top with the noodles. Sprinkle with sesame seeds, sliced avocado, and red pepper flakes (if using). Drizzle with the dressing and serve.

Leftovers Tip: Store the dressing, noodles, and greens separately in airtight containers and refrigerate. The noodles and greens will stay fresh for up to 3 days and the dressing for up to 1 week.

Per serving: Calories: 401; Fat: 15g; Carbohydrates: 60g; Protein: 13g; Fiber: 8g; Sodium: 536mg

LEMONY HERBED LENTIL SOUP

GLUTEN-FREE, NUT-FREE, SOY-FREE

PREP TIME: 10 minutes / **COOK TIME:** 35 minutes / **MAKES 2 SERVINGS**

Cozy, tasty, filling, and chock-full of nutrition, it's impossible to go wrong with lentil soup! To speed things up, you can drain 2 (15-ounce) cans of lentils and add them to the skillet with the celery, carrots, and potatoes instead of using dried.

1 cup dried brown or green
   lentils, rinsed

4 cups water

1 teaspoon extra-virgin olive oil

½ small yellow onion, chopped

2 garlic cloves, minced

1 celery stalk, minced

2 carrots, sliced

1 potato, peeled and diced

1 zucchini, diced

1 (15-ounce) can crushed
   tomatoes

1 teaspoon Italian seasoning

½ teaspoon smoked paprika

2 cups baby spinach

Juice of 1 lemon

1 teaspoon salt, plus more
   as needed

1. In a large saucepan, combine the lentils and water and bring to a boil over high heat. Lower the heat to medium and cook until soft, about 25 minutes.

2. Meanwhile, in a large skillet, heat the olive oil over medium heat. Add the onion and garlic and cook until fragrant, about 5 minutes. Add the celery, carrots, and potato and cook for 5 minutes. Add the mixture to the cooked lentils and stir until combined.

3. Add the zucchini, tomatoes, Italian seasoning, and smoked paprika and bring to a boil over medium-high heat. Lower the heat to medium and simmer until the flavors meld, about 10 minutes.

4. Add the spinach, stir, and cook until wilted. Add the lemon juice and salt and stir until combined. Taste and add more salt if needed.

Per serving: Calories: 546; Fat: 5g; Carbohydrates: 102g; Protein: 31g; Fiber: 21g; Sodium: 1,502mg

BROCCOLI AND "CHEDDAR" SOUP

GLUTEN-FREE, NUT-FREE, OIL-FREE

PREP TIME: 10 minutes / **COOK TIME:** 30 minutes / **MAKES 4 SERVINGS**

This soup is so delicious and cheezy that you will be double-checking the ingredients to make sure you didn't add real cheese by accident! Really quick, easy, and so tasty, it will blow your mind how similar in taste and texture this is to the old classic. It makes a filling weeknight dinner with a side salad or a lunch with some crusty bread so you can make sure you get every drop.

4 cups peeled and diced butternut squash

2 sweet potatoes, peeled and diced (about 2 cups)

1 small yellow onion, peeled and halved

2 garlic cloves, peeled

4 cups water

2 teaspoons salt

1 (13-ounce) can light unsweetened coconut milk

1 tablespoon red miso paste

3 tablespoons nutritional yeast

1 tablespoon tapioca flour

3 cups frozen broccoli

1. In a large pot, combine the butternut squash, sweet potatoes, onion, garlic, and water and bring to a boil over high heat. Lower the heat to medium-low and cook until fork-tender, about 20 minutes.

2. Transfer the mixture (including the liquid) to a blender and puree until smooth. You may need to do this in batches.

3. Return the soup to the pot and add the salt, coconut milk, red miso, nutritional yeast, tapioca flour, and broccoli and cook over medium heat, stirring often, until heated through, about 10 minutes.

Cooking Tip: For a smoother soup, use an immersion blender to break up the broccoli into smaller pieces or pulse the broccoli in a blender before adding it to the soup.

Per serving: Calories: 353; Fat: 20g; Carbohydrates: 42g; Protein: 8g; Fiber: 9g; Sodium: 1,404mg

SPLIT PEA AND SWEET POTATO SOUP

GLUTEN-FREE, NUT-FREE, SOY-FREE

PREP TIME: 5 minutes / **COOK TIME:** 40 minutes / **MAKES 4 SERVINGS**

This new-school version of a classic with sweet potatoes is über-creamy and absolutely delicious. No need to add ham—this soup is perfect without it.

---

2 cups dried split peas

1 tablespoon extra-virgin olive oil

2 garlic cloves, minced

1 small yellow onion, diced small

2 celery stalks, cut into ¼-inch pieces

2 large carrots, peeled and cut into ¼-inch pieces

1 teaspoon salt

2 sweet potatoes, peeled and cut into 1-inch pieces

1 teaspoon ground turmeric

1 teaspoon smoked paprika

1. Pour the split peas into a large pot and cover with water by 2 inches. Set the pot over high heat and bring to a boil, stirring often. Check the water level regularly and add more, if needed, so that there is always 2 inches above the peas. Cook until the peas break down and the soup looks like a very thick gravy, about 30 minutes.

2. Meanwhile, in a large skillet, heat the oil over medium heat. Add the garlic and onion and cook, stirring often, until fragrant, 3 to 5 minutes. Add the celery, carrots, and salt and cook, stirring often, for 5 minutes

3. Add the cooked vegetables, sweet potatoes, turmeric, and paprika to the pot and mix well. Cook, stirring often, until the sweet potatoes are fork-tender, about 10 minutes.

Cooking Tip: This recipe works well in an Instant Pot, which will reduce the time substantially. On the sauté mode, combine the oil, garlic, onion, celery, and carrots and cook for 5 minutes. Add the salt, sweet potatoes, split peas, turmeric, smoked paprika, and 6 cups of water. Seal the lid and pressure cook on high for 15 minutes. Let sit for 5 minutes before releasing the pressure.

Per serving: Calories: 462; Fat: 5g; Carbohydrates: 83g; Protein: 25g; Fiber: 29g; Sodium: 665mg

BEEFLESS IRISH STEW

PREP TIME: 10 minutes / **COOK TIME:** 30 minutes / **MAKES 4 SERVINGS**

Super filling thanks to the potatoes and peas yet easy on your digestion, you will love this stew. Pair it with some cooked quinoa, noodles, or rice for a heartier meal, or with a piece of crusty bread for mopping up the rich broth. If beer isn't your thing, just omit it; the dish will still be tasty.

- 1 teaspoon extra-virgin olive oil
- 1 small yellow onion, diced small
- 2 garlic cloves, minced
- 3 carrots, peeled, and cut into rounds
- 1 celery stalk, thinly sliced
- 1 cup stout or porter beer
- 1 (15-ounce) can crushed tomatoes
- 2 sweet potatoes, peeled and cut into cubes
- 4 small red potatoes, cut into cubes
- 5 cups water
- ½ cup frozen peas
- 1 teaspoon smoked paprika
- ½ teaspoon dried thyme
- 1 teaspoon salt
- ½ teaspoon black pepper

1. In a large pot, heat the olive oil over medium heat. Add the onion and garlic and cook, stirring often, until fragrant, about 5 minutes. Add the carrots and celery and cook, stirring often, for 5 more minutes.

2. Add the beer and bring to a boil. Cook for 3 minutes. Add the tomatoes, sweet potatoes, red potatoes, and water and stir until combined. Raise the heat to medium-high and bring to a boil.

3. Add the peas, smoked paprika, thyme, salt, and black pepper, lower the heat to medium, and simmer until the vegetables are fork-tender and the stew has thickened, about 20 minutes.

Variation Tip: Substitute 2 cups of cubed butternut squash for the sweet potatoes for an even richer broth.

Per serving: Calories: 272; Fat: 2g; Carbohydrates: 55g; Protein: 7g; Fiber: 10g; Sodium: 828mg

TOFU AND VEGETABLE FRIED RICE

NUT-FREE, ONE PAN, QUICK

PREP TIME: 10 minutes / **COOK TIME:** 15 minutes / **MAKES 4 SERVINGS**

Fried rice is the perfect quick and easy meal and a great way to use up leftover cooked rice and the odds and ends in your refrigerator. Substitute whatever vegetables you have on hand or tempeh or edamame for the tofu.

1 tablespoon sesame oil

1 (16-ounce) package extra-firm tofu, drained and diced small

1 bell pepper (any color), seeded and diced small

½ cup frozen peas

½ cup frozen corn

1 cup fresh or frozen broccoli florets

½ teaspoon garlic powder

2 tablespoons water

2 tablespoons low-sodium soy sauce or gluten-free tamari

1 tablespoon maple syrup

2 cups leftover cooked brown rice

1 scallion, white and green parts, thinly sliced, for garnish (optional)

1. In a wok or large skillet, heat the sesame oil over medium-high heat. Add the tofu and cook, stirring occasionally, until browned, about 5 minutes.

2. Add the bell pepper, peas, corn, broccoli, and garlic powder and cook, stirring often, for 5 minutes. Add the water to help soften the broccoli and cook until the liquid evaporates, about 3 minutes.

3. Add the soy sauce and maple syrup and mix well. Add the rice and cook until the rice is hot, 2 to 3 minutes. Spoon into bowls, garnish with the scallion (if using), and serve immediately.

Ingredient Tip: This works best with leftover cooked rice because it needs to be slightly dry to fry properly. Otherwise, it will stick to the pan and get a gummy texture.

Per serving: Calories: 319; Fat: 11g; Carbohydrates: 40g; Protein: 18g; Fiber: 5g; Sodium: 299mg

SPICED KIDNEY BEAN CURRY

GLUTEN-FREE, NUT-FREE, ONE PAN, QUICK, SOY-FREE

PREP TIME: 5 minutes / **COOK TIME:** 20 minutes / **MAKES 4 SERVINGS**

I love the texture of the meaty kidney beans paired with the spicy gravy in this scrumptious curry. Eat it in a bowl with half rice and half curry, topped with copious amounts of chopped cilantro and red pepper flakes. Or top a bowl with chopped cilantro, avocado, and onions and serve with soft bread on the side. It is like a brilliant Indian-inspired twist on chili, and no matter how you eat it, it is sure to be a hit.

1 teaspoon extra-virgin olive oil

2 garlic cloves, minced

2 teaspoons minced fresh ginger

1 small yellow onion, chopped small

2 (15-ounce) cans kidney beans, drained and rinsed

3 teaspoons curry powder

½ teaspoon salt

1 (15-ounce) can crushed tomatoes

2 cups water

4 generous tablespoons chopped fresh cilantro, for garnish

Red pepper flakes, for garnish (optional)

1. In a large saucepan or wok, heat the olive oil over medium heat. Add the garlic, ginger, and onion and cook until the onions are browned, about 7 minutes. Add the kidney beans, curry powder, salt, tomatoes, and water, raise the heat to high, and bring to a boil, stirring often.

2. Turn the heat to low and, using a potato masher, gently mash the ingredients to break up some of the beans, which will help thicken the curry, and simmer for 10 minutes. Spoon the curry into bowls, garnish with cilantro and red pepper flakes (if using), and serve.

Leftovers Tip: Refrigerate covered leftovers for up to 5 days or freeze for up to 3 months.

Per serving: Calories: 230; Fat: 2g; Carbohydrates: 42g; Protein: 14g; Fiber: 12g; Sodium: 505mg

BERBERE-SPICED RED LENTILS

GLUTEN-FREE, NUT-FREE, QUICK, SOY-FREE

PREP TIME: 5 minutes / **COOK TIME:** 25 minutes / **MAKES 4 SERVINGS**

If you have never tried Ethiopian food, you are in for a treat. Berbere spice is a seasoning blend that usually includes coriander, cumin, cardamom, dried chile peppers, nutmeg, ginger, turmeric, and cinnamon, plus many others. These lentils go great with a whole-grain pita and side of greens.

1 cup dried red lentils, rinsed

3 cups water

1 teaspoon extra-virgin olive oil

2 garlic cloves, minced

½ medium yellow onion, chopped small

3 tomatoes, chopped

2 tablespoons berbere spice

1 teaspoon salt

2 teaspoons tomato paste

1. In a large saucepan, combine the lentils and water over high heat and bring to a boil. Lower the heat to medium-low and cook, checking occasionally and adding more water if needed, for 20 minutes.

2. In a medium skillet, heat the olive oil over medium heat. Add the garlic and onion and cook until fragrant, 3 to 5 minutes

3. Add the tomatoes, berbere spice, salt, and tomato paste and cook, stirring constantly, until the mixture turns a deep red and becomes paste-like, about 5 minutes. Set aside.

4. Add the spiced tomato-and-onion mixture to the lentils and simmer over medium heat until the flavors combine and it's very thick, about 5 minutes. Serve immediately.

Ingredient Tip: Berbere spice is readily available in the spice aisle of most super-markets. If you can't find it, mix together 1 teaspoon smoked paprika, ½ teaspoon cayenne pepper, ¼ teaspoon coriander, and ¼ teaspoon cinnamon.

Per serving: Calories: 216; Fat: 3g; Carbohydrates: 38g; Protein: 13g; Fiber: 8g; Sodium: 594mg

LAZY LASAGNA BAKED ZITI

PREP TIME: 10 minutes / **COOK TIME:** 30 minutes / **MAKES 4 SERVINGS**

This recipe makes it possible to have that home-cooked lasagna experience in a fraction of the time. The tofu mimics ricotta, and the Nutty Plant-Based Parmesan (page 174) gives such an umami punch that you'll have to remind yourself there's no actual cheese in the dish. To make this even faster, use store-bought marinara instead of making your own. This will cut out quite a bit of prep and cook time and make the assembly a breeze.

1 pound whole-wheat ziti pasta

FOR THE SAUCE

1 teaspoon extra-virgin olive oil

2 garlic cloves, minced

½ medium yellow onion, diced small

1 red or yellow bell pepper, roughly chopped

1 (28-ounce) can crushed tomatoes

1 teaspoon Italian seasoning

Pinch red pepper flakes

½ teaspoon salt

1 teaspoon maple syrup

1 cup water

FOR THE RICOTTA

1 (16-ounce) package extra-firm tofu, drained

2 tablespoons nutritional yeast

1 teaspoon salt

1 tablespoon tapioca flour

1 teaspoon Italian seasoning

FOR SERVING

2 tablespoons chopped fresh basil

¼ cup store-bought plant-based Parmesan or Nutty Plant-Based Parmesan (page 174) (optional)

1. Preheat the oven to 375°F.

2. Bring a large pot of water to a boil over high heat. Add the pasta and cook according to the package instructions. Drain and set aside.

3. **Make the sauce:** While the pasta is cooking, in a saucepan, heat the olive oil over medium heat. Add the garlic, onion, and bell pepper and cook, stirring often, until fragrant, about 5 minutes. Add the crushed tomatoes, Italian seasoning, red pepper flakes, salt, maple syrup, and water and bring to a boil. Lower the heat to medium-low and simmer for 5 minutes. Set aside 2 cups of sauce; store the rest in an airtight container and refrigerate for up to 5 days or freeze for up to 3 months.

4. **Make the ricotta:** In a medium bowl, combine the tofu, nutritional yeast, salt, tapioca flour, and Italian seasoning and, using your hands, break up the tofu and mix until well incorporated.

5. **Assemble the dish:** In a large 8-by-12-inch baking dish, combine the cooked pasta and the reserved 2 cups of sauce. (You can use more or less sauce depending on your preferences.) Crumble the ricotta mixture over the pasta and fold gently into the pasta, leaving pockets of cheeziness; do not completely mix everything together.

6. Cover the baking dish with aluminum foil and bake for 15 minutes, or until it is hot and steaming in the center. Spoon into shallow bowls and garnish with fresh basil and plant-based Parmesan (if using).

Variation Tip: For a less gluten-heavy meal, add 16 ounces of frozen cauliflower florets to the sauce and reduce the amount of pasta by half. Another option is to add 2 cups of baby spinach to the sauce and mix until wilted before stirring it into the pasta.

Per serving: Calories: 613; Fat: 10g; Carbohydrates: 109g; Protein: 34g; Fiber: 14g; Sodium: 1,319mg

CREAMY FRUIT SALAD

GLUTEN-FREE, NO COOK, OIL-FREE, QUICK

PREP TIME: 15 minutes / **MAKES 4 SERVINGS**

This unusual fruit salad is inspired by one I had at many Mexican Christmas parties that I attended during the years I lived in California. The more traditional dish includes sour cream or condensed milk, but I substitute plant-based yogurt with great results. This salad is best when it rests for a few hours to give the flavors time to meld, so prepare it early and store in the fridge until dessert.

4 red apples, any kind, cored and diced

1 (15-ounce) can pineapple chunks, drained, or 2 cups fresh pineapple chunks

¼ cup raisins

¼ cup chopped pecans or walnuts

1 cup plain plant-based yogurt

2 teaspoons maple syrup

In a large bowl, combine the apples and pineapples and toss well to make sure the apples are covered in pineapple juice to prevent browning. Add the raisins, nuts, yogurt, and maple syrup and mix well. Cover and refrigerate for at least 2 hours to develop the flavors.

Leftovers Tip: Refrigerate leftovers for up to 2 days.

Variation Tip: Make this a bit more savory by omitting the maple syrup and adding 1 stalk chopped celery, 1 peeled and chopped carrot, and a pinch of salt.

Per serving (1½ cups): Calories: 267; Fat: 5g; Carbohydrates: 54g; Protein: 6g; Fiber: 6g; Sodium: 52mg

ACAI AND GRANOLA SMOOTHIE BOWLS

NO COOK, OIL-FREE, QUICK

PREP TIME: 10 minutes / **MAKES 2 SERVINGS**

This superfood smoothie tastes great with whatever liquids or frozen fruits you have on hand. The only rules are to use frozen bananas and frozen acai, and not to add too much liquid. Beautifully colored and antioxidant-rich, acai doesn't have much flavor, so adding fruit juice or frozen fruit is a must. Peel and cut the bananas into 2-inch slices and freeze the night before.

2 frozen sliced bananas

2 (3½-ounce) frozen acai packets, broken into pieces

1 cup frozen strawberries

¾ cup unsweetened plant-based milk

2 tablespoons nut butter

½ cup store-bought granola or Crispy, Crunchy Granola (page 184)

2 tablespoons chia seeds

2 tablespoons cacao nibs

½ cup chopped fresh pineapple or canned no-sugar-added diced pineapple, drained

1. In a blender, combine the frozen banana, acai, strawberries, and about half of the plant-based milk and blend for 1 minute. Scrape down the sides of the blender, add the remaining plant-based milk, and blend again. You may need to scrape down the sides of the blender one or two more times until the acai and fruit blends well.

2. Divide the mixture between 2 bowls and arrange the nut butter, granola, chia seeds, cacao nibs, and pineapple in a decorative pattern over each smoothie.

Ingredient Tip: Packages of acai are available in the freezer section of most supermarkets. Or use 1 cup of another chopped frozen fruit.

Per serving: Calories: 566; Fat: 26g; Carbohydrates: 75g; Protein: 13g; Fiber: 16g; Sodium: 112mg

PEANUT BUTTER COOKIES

OIL-FREE, QUICK, SOY-FREE

PREP TIME: 10 minutes / **COOK TIME:** 13 minutes / **MAKES 10 COOKIES**

Peanut butter is amazing in all forms, and these treats are a delicious way to use it. They might be the easiest and quickest cookies you will ever make. They have only a hint of sweetness, but they are full of that peanut-y goodness we all adore.

2 tablespoons ground flaxseeds

6 tablespoons cold water

¼ cup maple syrup

1 tablespoon baking powder

1 cup natural peanut butter

½ cup whole-wheat flour

1. Preheat the oven to 350°F. Line a sheet pan with parchment paper.

2. In a large bowl, mix together the ground flaxseeds and water to make "flax eggs" and let sit until it gels, about 10 minutes.

3. Add the maple syrup, baking powder, peanut butter, and flour to the bowl and mix well with a fork.

4. Put rounded tablespoons of the batter onto the prepared sheet pan. Flatten each cookie and, using the back of a fork, press a crisscross pattern into each one. Bake for 13 to 15 minutes, or until they are firm and slightly golden.

Leftovers Tip: Store the cookies in an airtight container and keep at room temperature for up to 4 days.

Variation Tip: If you love the combo of chocolate and peanut butter like most people do, add ½ cup vegan refined-sugar-free chocolate-chunks to the recipe. If you want to really go for it, stir in ½ cup of broken pretzels, too!

Per serving (2 cookies): Calories: 409; Fat: 28g; Carbohydrates: 33g; Protein: 14g; Fiber: 5g; Sodium: 14mg

COCONUT AND TAHINI BLISS BALLS

NO COOK, OIL-FREE, QUICK

PREP TIME: 10 minutes / **MAKES 9 BALLS**

Bliss balls, sometimes called energy balls, are one of the most convenient, decadent-yet-healthy treats around. With a texture reminiscent of cookie dough, they are super scrumptious while still packing a serious protein and fiber punch! They're easy to make and so versatile, you'll become a bliss ball aficionado in no time. See the Variation Tip below for a couple of my favorite variations.

½ cup cashews

½ cups walnuts

½ cup rolled oats

2 tablespoons maple syrup

3 tablespoons sesame tahini

½ cup unsweetened shredded coconut, divided

1. In a blender, pulse the cashews and walnuts until you have a combination of smaller pieces and nut dust. Transfer the mixture to a medium bowl and add the oats, maple syrup, tahini, and ¼ cup of coconut and mix well. The mixture will be sticky.

2. Put the remaining coconut on a plate. Roll the mixture into 9 equal-size balls. Roll each ball in the coconut until evenly coated. Some will stick, some won't. It will only be a thin layer of coconut coating.

3. Set the finished balls on a sheet pan or plate and refrigerate for at least 30 minutes to set. Eat immediately or store in an airtight container and refrigerate for up to 7 days.

Variation Tip: Omit the tahini and use peanut butter. Roll the balls in unsweetened cocoa powder for a delicious peanut butter and chocolate treat. Or omit the maple syrup and add 5 pitted dates to the food processor along with the nuts. This will make a stickier bliss ball with a more subtle sweetness.

Per serving (3 balls): Calories: 419; Fat: 32g; Carbohydrates: 29g; Protein: 10g; Fiber: 6g; Sodium: 24mg

VANILLA NICE CREAM

5 INGREDIENTS, GLUTEN-FREE, NO COOK, NUT-FREE, OIL-FREE, QUICK

PREP TIME: 5 minutes / **MAKES 2 SERVINGS**

Nice cream, a super-easy plant-based ice cream, is made from blending frozen bananas with a tiny bit of liquid and other flavorings. The result is unbelievably creamy and so versatile that it pairs well with everything from strawberries to cinnamon (see the Variation Tip below). Be sure to peel the bananas and cut them into 2-inch slices before freezing for the easiest prep.

2 frozen sliced bananas

½ teaspoon vanilla extract

3 tablespoons unsweetened plant-based milk

1 teaspoon maple syrup

1. In a food processor or high-speed blender, combine the bananas, vanilla, plant-based milk, and maple syrup and blend until smooth and creamy. You will have to stop the machine to scrape down the sides two or three times before the desired consistency of soft-serve ice cream is achieved.

2. Serve immediately or store in an airtight container and freeze for later. Be sure to pull it out of the freezer 10 to 15 minutes before you want to serve it to let it soften. Otherwise, it will be hard to scoop.

Variation Tip: For chocolate nice cream, omit the vanilla and add 2 tablespoons of unsweetened cocoa powder and 1 additional teaspoon of maple syrup. For strawberry nice cream, omit the vanilla and add 1 cup frozen strawberries and an additional 2 tablespoons of plant-based milk.

Per serving (½ cup): Calories: 130; Fat: 1g; Carbohydrates: 30g; Protein: 2g; Fiber: 3g; Sodium: 11mg

SUPER-SIMPLE GUACAMOLE

PREP TIME: 10 minutes / **MAKES ABOUT 1½ CUPS**

A go-to guac is a must-have in anyone's recipe repertoire, and this one will knock your socks off with its flavor. With an ingredient as perfect as a ripe, buttery avocado, it's best to keep it simple so you can enhance but not over-power it. I like to keep my guacamole mild and save the spice for salsa, but if you like your guac with a kick, stir in a chopped jalapeño.

2 avocados, peeled and pitted

Juice of ½ lime

Pinch salt

2 tablespoons chopped fresh cilantro

1 tomato, chopped

1 scallion, white and green parts, chopped

In a medium bowl, combine the avocados, lime juice, and salt and mash together until it reaches your desired consistency. Add the cilantro, tomato, and scallion and mix well. Serve immediately.

Leftovers Tip: Avocados turns brown when exposed to air, just like apples and bananas. The best way to combat this is to make a physical barrier using plastic wrap so air cannot get in. Press the plastic wrap gently directly onto the guacamole. This is only pertinent when making a double or triple batch because, let's face it, having leftovers is seldom a reality.

Per serving (¼ cup): Calories: 113; Fat: 10g; Carbohydrates: 7g; Protein: 2g; Fiber: 5g; Sodium: 32mg

PICO DE GALLO

5 INGREDIENTS, GLUTEN-FREE, NO COOK, NUT-FREE, OIL-FREE, ONE BOWL, QUICK, SOY-FREE

PREP TIME: 15 minutes / **MAKES 2 CUPS**

Pico de gallo is one of the freshest and healthiest condiments around, especially when you can get your hands on super-ripe red tomatoes. I love the tang of the lime juice paired with the tomatoes, onions, and jalapeños, and the cilantro gives it just the right zing. Whether you pair it with chips or add it to the Pulled Jackfruit Tacos (page 119) or the Black Bean Tortas (page 149), this salsa will be the life of the party.

4 tomatoes, chopped small

1 medium yellow onion, minced

1 jalapeño pepper, seeded
   and minced

Juice of 1 lime, plus more
   if needed

Pinch salt, plus more if needed

3 tablespoons chopped fresh
   cilantro

In a large bowl, mix together the tomatoes, onion, jalapeño, lime juice, salt, and cilantro. Taste and adjust seasoning if desired. The salsa can be stored in an airtight container in the refrigerator for up to 4 days.

Variation Tip: Turn your pico de gallo into a tangy mango salsa by peeling and chopping up a ripe mango and mixing it in! This is a great option for topping a veggie burger or some grilled tofu.

Per serving (¼ cup): Calories: 19; Fat: 0g; Carbohydrates: 4g; Protein: 1g; Fiber: 1g; Sodium: 23mg

JALAPEÑO AND TOMATILLO SALSA

5 INGREDIENTS, GLUTEN-FREE, NO COOK, NUT-FREE,
OIL-FREE, QUICK, SOY-FREE

PREP TIME: 10 minutes / **MAKES ABOUT 3 CUPS**

There are few meals that I think won't be improved with some heat, whether from a dash of hot sauce, a pinch of red pepper flakes, or a spoonful of spicy salsa. This recipe uses raw tomatillos and jalapeños, which gives the salsa a super-fresh kick that is perfect with Pulled Jackfruit Tacos (page 119), Tofu Rancheros (page 110), and Black Bean and Quinoa Burrito Bowls (page 93). Some jalapeños are hotter than others, so play around with the amount to get your desired heat level.

4 tomatillos, peeled and washed

3 jalapeño peppers, stemmed and seeded

½ medium yellow onion, peeled

1 garlic clove

½ bunch fresh cilantro (about 1 cup leaves and stems)

¼ teaspoon salt, plus more as needed

1 cup water

In a blender, combine the tomatillos, jalapeños, onion, garlic, cilantro, salt, and water and blend until smooth. Taste and add salt if desired. Store in an airtight container in the refrigerator for up to 10 days.

Ingredient Tip: Tomatillos are small, tart, green tomato-like fruits that are covered with a papery husk. Select larger ones, if you can find them, that are free from black spots. It is normal for them to feel sticky when you remove the husks, but they shouldn't feel slimy. Wash them well with warm water to remove the sticky substance. If needed, you can substitute 3 Roma tomatoes, but note that the flavor and color of the salsa will be different.

Variation Tip: If you like a mellower roasted salsa flavor, you can roast the tomatillos, jalapeños, onion, and garlic on an oiled sheet pan for 20 minutes in a 400°F oven. Finish by blending the roasted vegetables with the cilantro, salt, and water and let cool thoroughly before storing.

Per serving (¼ cup): Calories: 7; Fat: 0g; Carbohydrates: 1g; Protein: 0g; Fiber: 0g; Sodium: 50mg

NUTTY PLANT-BASED PARMESAN

5 INGREDIENTS, GLUTEN-FREE, NO COOK, OIL-FREE, QUICK, SOY-FREE

PREP TIME: 10 minutes / **MAKES 1½ CUPS**

This plant-based substitute for Parmesan cheese is so good, it's nutty. Pun intended. And with only three ingredients, you can whip it up in a flash. You'll be shocked at how similar in taste and texture it is to grated Parmesan cheese! It is wonderful sprinkled on Lentil Bolognese (page 96), Fettuccine with Creamy Cashew Alfredo (page 66), or Meatless Meatballs with Quick Marinara Sauce (page 122). However, if you have a sensitivity to MSG, beware—you may find yourself having a similar reaction because nutritional yeast has some naturally occurring MSG present. Severe reactions are not very common, but if you have doubts, consult your doctor first.

---

1 cup raw cashews
½ cup nutritional yeast

½ teaspoon salt

In a blender, pulse the cashews until they become a fine dust. Transfer the cashew dust to a small bowl and add the nutritional yeast and salt. Mix well with a spoon. Transfer any leftovers to an airtight container and refrigerate for up to 10 days or freeze for up to 3 months.

Per serving (2 tablespoons): Calories: 79; Fat: 5g; Carbohydrates: 5g; Protein: 3g; Fiber: 0g; Sodium: 195mg

NUT MILK

5 INGREDIENTS, GLUTEN-FREE, NO COOK, OIL-FREE, SOY-FREE

PREP TIME: 5 minutes, plus overnight to soak / **MAKES 5 CUPS**

Making your own nut milk is easy, and it was a total game changer when I learned that it needed minimal ingredients and equipment. Simply soak nuts overnight when your milk supply is getting low, and you can make a new batch in a jiff the next day. I like to make mine without the dates or vanilla, because then I can use the milk in savory preparations like Quick Creamy Herbed Tomato Soup (page 36) and Broccoli and "Cheddar" Soup (page 158), but if you prefer a sweeter milk, add them.

1 cup raw cashews or almonds, soaked overnight and drained

3 dates, pitted (optional)

1 teaspoon vanilla extract (optional)

4 cups water

1. In a blender combine the soaked nuts, dates (if using), vanilla (if using), and water and blend on high for 3 to 4 minutes, until the nuts are all pulverized and the liquid looks creamy.

2. Pour the blended mix through a nut milk bag, cheesecloth, or a fine-mesh sieve and pour it into an airtight storage container. Chill and use within 4 days.

Ingredient Tip: If you forget to soak the nuts, you can boil them in water for 20 minutes. Soaking them overnight is ideal, though, because it makes a creamier milk.

Per serving (1 cup): Calories: 25; Fat: 2g; Carbohydrates: 1g; Protein: 0g; Fiber: 0g; Sodium: 22mg

OAT MILK

PREP TIME: 5 minutes / **MAKES 4 CUPS**

Oat milk is one of the creamiest and most versatile of the plant-based milks, and I find it most closely mimics cow's milk. Plus, there is zero soaking needed, so it's great for those last-minute milk emergencies. I like to use it in the Plant-Based Queso Dip (page 139) and Plant-Based Mango Lassi Smoothies (page 136).

1 cup rolled oats   **4 cups water**
3 dates, pitted (optional)

1. In a blender, combine the oats, dates (if using), and water and blend on high for 45 seconds, until the oats are pulverized and the liquid looks creamy. Be careful not to overblend, as the texture will become slimy and unpleasant.

2. Pour the mixture through a nut milk bag, cheesecloth, or fine-mesh sieve to strain out all the small pieces. Pour it into an airtight storage container and chill for up to 4 days.

> **Variation Tip:** To make strawberry oat milk, first add 1 cup sliced strawberries and the water to the blender and blend until smooth. Add the oats, blend for 45 seconds, and then strain.

Per serving (1 cup): Calories: 90; Fat: 3g; Carbohydrates: 13g; Protein: 1g; Fiber: 0g; Sodium: 12mg

SPICY ITALIAN VINAIGRETTE

5 INGREDIENTS, GLUTEN-FREE, NO COOK, NUT-FREE, QUICK, SOY-FREE

PREP TIME: 5 minutes / **MAKES 1 CUP**

I am truly a salad fiend. A quick look at my Instagram or blog will show you that salad is one of my specialties. Almost as important as what you put *in* a salad is what you put *on* it. A traditional vinaigrette, with a ratio of 3:1 oil to vinegar, is a bit oily for my tastes; I prefer a 2:1 ratio, resulting in a healthier dressing with a bigger burst of vinegary flavor. This is so good you'll want to mop up the extra with some crusty bread, but keep in mind that a little goes a long way.

1 cup apple cider vinegar

½ cup extra-virgin olive oil

2 teaspoons maple syrup

2 teaspoons Italian seasoning

¼ teaspoon salt

¼ teaspoon black pepper

½ teaspoon garlic powder

Pinch red pepper flakes

Combine the apple cider vinegar, olive oil, maple syrup, Italian seasoning, salt, black pepper, garlic powder, and red pepper flakes in a jar, cover, and shake until well blended. The dressing can be stored in the refrigerator for up to 2 weeks.

Variation Tip: If you prefer a more emulsified vinaigrette, prepare it as follows: In a wide mouth jar, combine the vinegar, maple syrup, salt, and garlic powder and blend with an immersion blender. Add the Italian seasoning, black pepper, and red pepper flakes. With the immersion blender running, slowly pour in the olive oil until a creamy consistency is achieved.

Per serving (2 tablespoons): Calories: 131; Fat: 14g; Carbohydrates: 2g; Protein: 0g; Fiber: 0g; Sodium: 75mg

PLANT-BASED MAYO 3 WAYS

5 INGREDIENTS, GLUTEN-FREE, NO COOK, NUT-FREE, ONE BOWL, QUICK, SOY-FREE

PREP TIME: 10 minutes / **MAKES 1 CUP**

The only thing that stands between you and easy homemade mayo is an immersion blender, which is the best way to achieve consistent results. These three versions are perfect for sandwiches like the Brown Rice and Black Bean Veggie Burgers (page 34) or as a dip for some nibbly treats. Once you get the technique down, the sky is the limit: experiment with adding gochujang or wasabi to spice up your life. The secret ingredient to make this plant-based is aquafaba, the liquid you usually drain and discard from a can of chickpeas. Next time you make a batch of Crispy Baked Chickpeas (page 146), save the aquafaba and make some mayo!

BASIC MAYO

¼ cup aquafaba

1 teaspoon apple cider vinegar

1 teaspoon Dijon mustard

1 tablespoon maple syrup

¼ teaspoon salt

¾ cup extra-virgin olive oil

ZESTY AVOCADO MAYO

¼ cup aquafaba

2 teaspoons Dijon mustard

Juice of 1 lime

1 tablespoon maple syrup

¼ teaspoon salt

1 ripe avocado, peeled and pitted

¾ cup extra-virgin olive oil

GARLIC AND HERB AIOLI

¼ cup aquafaba

1 tablespoon Dijon mustard

2 teaspoons apple cider vinegar

1 tablespoon maple syrup

¼ teaspoon salt

1 garlic clove, peeled

2 tablespoons chopped fresh herbs, like mint, cilantro, and/ or thyme

¾ cup extra-virgin olive oil

1. Combine all the ingredients for your desired mayo except the olive oil into a wide-mouthed jar. Using an immersion blender, blend until well combined and the mixture starts to thicken.

2. Add the olive oil, pouring it in slowly while the immersion blender is running. The liquid will start to grow in volume as the oil and aquafaba emulsify and bind.

3. The mayo is ready when the mixture reaches a thick consistency, 3 to 5 minutes. If the texture is not thick enough, add more olive oil, 1 tablespoon at a time, until it reaches the desired texture and thickness.

Leftovers Tip: Refrigerate, covered, for up to 5 days. Some separation is normal—simply reblend with an immersion blender or whisk with a fork.

Basic Mayo per serving (1 tablespoon): Calories: 93; Fat: 10g; Carbohydrates: 1g; Protein: 0g; Fiber: 0g; Sodium: 40mg

Zesty Avocado Mayo per serving (1 tablespoon): Calories: 114; Fat: 12g; Carbohydrates: 2g; Protein: 0g; Fiber: 1g; Sodium: 41mg

Garlic and Herb Aioli per serving (1 tablespoon): Calories: 93; Fat: 10g; Carbohydrates: 1g; Protein: 0g; Fiber: 0g; Sodium: 40mg

SUGAR-FREE KETCHUP

PREP TIME: 5 minutes / **COOK TIME:** 20 minutes / **MAKES 2 CUPS**

Most ketchup you can find at your grocery store is loaded with added sugar, but this super-simple recipe is a way to give your staple condiment a WFPB makeover. Keep in mind that it will not be as sweet as you're used to, but it captures the essence of classic ketchup, and with enough time, your taste buds will adjust. Add your favorite hot sauce for an extra kick or some plant-based buffalo sauce to make a great coating for baked tofu!

1 (15-ounce) can tomato sauce

3 tablespoons apple cider vinegar

3 tablespoons maple syrup

½ teaspoon salt

1 teaspoon onion powder

1 teaspoon garlic powder

2 tablespoons tomato paste

1. In a medium saucepan, combine the tomato sauce, vinegar, maple syrup, salt, onion powder, garlic powder, and tomato paste and bring to a boil over medium-high heat.

2. Lower the heat to medium-low and simmer, stirring often, for 20 minutes. Let cool and store in an airtight container in the refrigerator for up to 10 days.

Per serving (2 tablespoons): Calories: 20; Fat: 0g; Carbohydrates: 5g; Protein: 0g; Fiber: 1g; Sodium: 201mg

BBQ SAUCE

GLUTEN-FREE, NUT-FREE, OIL-FREE, ONE PAN, QUICK, SOY-FREE

COOK TIME: 20 minutes / **MAKES 1½ CUPS**

In this recipe I use blackstrap molasses instead of refined sugar for sweetness. Although it is a by-product of the sugar-refining process, its high calcium, iron, and magnesium content make it a vegan superfood, and I consciously choose to add it into my diet in moderation. If you object, feel free to substitute maple syrup or Raw Date Paste (page 183), but the sauce won't have the same depth of flavor or gorgeous color. Try this in BBQ Tempeh Succotash Skillet (page 120) or BBQ Jackfruit Sandwiches (page 152).

---

1 (15-ounce) can tomato sauce

¼ cup apple cider vinegar

3 tablespoons maple syrup

1 tablespoon blackstrap molasses or maple syrup

½ teaspoon salt

Pinch red pepper flakes

2 teaspoons onion powder

1 teaspoon garlic powder

2 tablespoons tomato paste

1 teaspoon smoked paprika

1. In a medium saucepan, combine the tomato sauce, apple cider vinegar, maple syrup, molasses, salt, red pepper flakes, onion powder, garlic powder, tomato paste, and smoked paprika and bring the mixture to a boil over medium-high heat.

2. Lower the heat to medium-low and simmer, stirring often, for 20 minutes. Let cool and store in an airtight container in the refrigerator for up to 10 days.

Per serving (2 tablespoons): Calories: 32; Fat: 0g; Carbohydrates: 8g; Protein: 1g; Fiber: 1g; Sodium: 269mg

STRAWBERRY CHIA JAM

5 INGREDIENTS, GLUTEN-FREE, NUT-FREE, OIL-FREE, QUICK, SOY-FREE

PREP TIME: 2 minutes / **COOK TIME:** 10 minutes / **MAKES 1½ CUPS**

This homemade jam is so easy to make you will wonder why you ever spent your money on a store-bought version. It's very much in demand at my house; my kids ask for it almost every week. I love that it's refined-sugar-free and sweetened with only dates, which are high in fiber, antioxidants, and iron. We enjoy this jam spread on toast, added to Peanut Butter and Strawberry Jam Oatmeal (page 29), or in a yogurt bowl or smoothies.

3 cups frozen strawberries

4 dates, pitted and chopped small

¼ cup water

3 tablespoons chia seeds

1. In a medium saucepan over medium-high heat, combine the strawberries, dates, and water and bring to a boil. Lower the heat to medium-low and simmer, stirring occasionally, for 10 minutes. Remove from the heat.

2. Using a potato masher, mash the mixture until the jam is smooth but with some chunks remaining. Add the chia seeds and stir well. Transfer the mixture to a small jar, cover, and let cool. The jam will thicken as it cools. The jam can be stored in the refrigerator for up to 5 days.

Variation Tip: Vary the recipe by using your favorite fresh or frozen fruits, such as peaches, apricots, blueberries, or a combination.

Per serving (2 tablespoons): Calories: 43; Fat: 1g; Carbohydrates: 8g; Protein: 1g; Fiber: 3g; Sodium: 2mg

RAW DATE PASTE

5 INGREDIENTS, GLUTEN-FREE, NO COOK, NUT-FREE, OIL-FREE, QUICK, SOY-FREE

PREP TIME: 10 minutes / **MAKES 2½ CUPS**

Dates are a delicious natural sweetener, and this raw date paste works really well to sweeten things up. Go ahead and substitute it for maple syrup in any recipe in this book, like the Sugar-Free Ketchup (page 180) or Peaches and Cream Overnight Oats (page 82). It will impart a darker hue to the recipes, since maple syrup is much lighter in color, and the sweetness will be subtler than maple syrup's. It is ideal for people who do not like things very sweet.

---

1 cup Medjool dates, pitted and chopped
1½ cups water

In a blender, combine the dates and water and blend until smooth. Store in an airtight container in the refrigerator for up to 7 days.

Per serving (2 tablespoons): Calories: 21; Fat: 0g; Carbohydrates: 5g; Protein: 0g; Fiber: 1g; Sodium: 0mg

CRISPY, CRUNCHY GRANOLA

PREP TIME: 5 minutes / **COOK TIME:** 20 minutes / **MAKES 4 CUPS**

I love the ease and versatility of homemade granola. Many times, I bust out a batch before I have even decided what will go into my smoothie bowl. It's tasty, crunchy, and it'll save you tons of money—commercial granolas are pricy! Even better, this recipe also has less oil and sugar than store-bought versions. Use it in Strawberry, Banana, and Granola Yogurt Bowls (page 32) or Blueberry and Peanut Butter Parfait Bowls (page 55).

3 cups rolled oats

¼ cup extra-virgin olive oil

¼ cup maple syrup

½ teaspoon salt

1 tablespoon pumpkin pie spice

½ cup chopped pecans

½ cup raisins

1. Preheat the oven to 350°F. Line a sheet pan with parchment paper.

2. In a large bowl mix together the oats, olive oil, and maple syrup and stir well until the oats are slightly wet. Add the salt and pumpkin pie spice and stir well.

3. Spread out the mixture gently on the sheet pan. It's okay if it's clumpy (granola clusters are delicious!). Bake for 10 minutes. Stir gently, being careful not to break up the clusters. Sprinkle the pecans on top and bake for another 10 minutes, or until it is golden and smells amazing. Since oven temperatures vary, if the granola is not ready, continue to bake and check every 2 minutes so the granola does not burn.

4. Let the granola cool completely. Add the raisins and stir gently until combined. Store the granola in an airtight container at room temperature for up to 2 weeks.

Variation Tip: For a super-nutty granola, add 3 tablespoons of peanut butter to the oat mixture in step 2. For a berry granola, omit the pumpkin pie spice and replace the raisins with dried berries. For a tropical take, omit the pumpkin pie spice, pecans, and raisins. Add ½ cup unsweetened coconut flakes to the oat mixture, and add ½ cup macadamia nut pieces halfway through the baking time. Then stir in ¼ cup of chopped dried mangoes after baking.

Per serving (¼ cup): Calories: 138; Fat: 7g; Carbohydrates: 18g; Protein: 3g; Fiber: 2g; Sodium: 74mg

REFERENCES

Active Times. "Is the Standard American Diet Making You Sad, Sick, and Tired?" April 18, 2018.

"Food's Carbon Footprint." GreenEatz.com/foods-carbon-footprint.html.

Harvard T. H. Chan School of Public Health. "The Nutrition Source: Straight Talk about Soy."

Holleman, Joey. "USC Study Finds Vegan Diet Most Effective at Weight Loss." University of South Carolina Arnold School of Public Health. November 10, 2014.

International Vegetarian Union Science Group. "What Every Vegan Should Know About Vitamin B12." Vegan Society. October 2001.

Kubala, Jillian, MS, RD. "Essential Amino Acids: Definition, Benefits and Food Sources." Healthline. June 12, 2018.

Landsverk, Gabby. "How Going Vegan Can Affect Your Body and Brain." Insider. October 10, 2019.

Lara, Kyla, MD. "Plant Based Diet Associated with Less Heart Failure Risk." American Heart Association. November 13, 2017.

Physicians Committee for Responsible Medicine. "Alzheimer's Disease: Boost Brain Health with a Plant-Based Diet."

———. "Food and Mood: Eating Plants to Fight the Blues." June 23, 2015.

———. "Heart Disease: Boost Heart Health with a Plant-Based Diet."

———. "Protein Power Up with Plant-Based Protein."

Tuso, Philip J., MD, Mohamed H. Ismail, MD, Benjamin P. Ha, MD, and Carole Bartolotto, MA, RD. "Nutritional Update for Physicians: Plant-Based Diets." *Permanente Journal* 17, no. 2 (Spring 2013): 61–66.

Winston, J. Craig, and Ann Reed Mangels. "Position of the American Dietetic Association: Vegetarian Diets." *Journal of the American Dietetic Association* 109, no. 7 (July 2009): 1266–82.

Zheng, Ju-Sheng, Stephen J. Sharp, Fumiaki Imamura, Rajiv Chowdhury et al. "Association of Plasma Biomarkers of Fruit and Vegetable Intake with Incident Type 2 Diabetes: EPIC-InterAct Case-Cohort Study in Eight European Countries." *BMJ* 2020 (July 8, 2020): 370.

MEASUREMENT CONVERSIONS

	US STANDARD	US STANDARD (OUNCES)	METRIC (APPROXIMATE)
VOLUME EQUIVALENTS (LIQUID)	2 tablespoons	1 fl. oz.	30 mL
	¼ cup	2 fl. oz.	60 mL
	½ cup	4 fl. oz.	120 mL
	1 cup	8 fl. oz.	240 mL
	1½ cups	12 fl. oz.	355 mL
	2 cups or 1 pint	16 fl. oz.	475 mL
	4 cups or 1 quart	32 fl. oz.	1 L
	1 gallon	128 fl. oz.	4 L
VOLUME EQUIVALENTS (DRY)	⅛ teaspoon	———	0.5 mL
	¼ teaspoon	———	1 mL
	½ teaspoon	———	2 mL
	¾ teaspoon	———	4 mL
	1 teaspoon	———	5 mL
	1 tablespoon	———	15 mL
	¼ cup	———	59 mL
	⅓ cup	———	79 mL
	½ cup	———	118 mL
	⅔ cup	———	156 mL
	¾ cup	———	177 mL
	1 cup	———	235 mL
	2 cups or 1 pint	———	475 mL
	3 cups	———	700 mL
	4 cups or 1 quart	———	1 L
	½ gallon	———	2 L
	1 gallon	———	4 L
WEIGHT EQUIVALENTS	½ ounce	———	15 g
	1 ounce	———	30 g
	2 ounces	———	60 g
	4 ounces	———	115 g
	8 ounces	———	225 g
	12 ounces	———	340 g
	16 ounces or 1 pound	———	455 g

	FAHRENHEIT (F)	CELSIUS (C) (APPROXIMATE)
OVEN TEMPERATURES	250°F	120°C
	300°F	150°C
	325°F	180°C
	375°F	190°C
	400°F	200°C
	425°F	220°C
	450°F	230°C

INDEX

ACKNOWLEDGMENTS

I thank:

My husband, David Tercero-Lopez, for tirelessly entertaining our kids, being my cheerful sous chef, testing recipes without complaint, and for tolerating my incessant chatter about food. Thank you for all your help, support, patience, and for going vegan with me. Our children, Mia, Ezra, and Alexa, for inspiring me to seek better health and vitality. My mother, Kathy Morrissey, and late grandmother Patricia Stone, for praising my healthy appetite and teaching me to cook confidently. My sister, Lauren O'Brien, for believing in me. My late fathers, Dennis Morrissey and Jim Maggio, for sharing their love of food. My influences and friends— Marilyn, Butterfield Kitchen, Roomies from 1993 to 2005, my Mikes, Jens, Sarahs, and Jess. Eric, Janice, Heidi, the Rudy's guys, and Bunmie. My editor, Gleni. My brother-in-law, Kevin O'Brien, for his technological know-how. My Instagram family, with extra gratitude to Kate Friedman of @herbivoreskitchen.

ABOUT THE AUTHOR

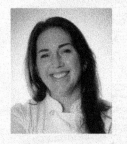

Sara Tercero is the face behind the popular blog *Better Food Guru*. She has cooked professionally for two decades and uses that expertise to create and share easy, health-conscious, and tasty recipes that anyone can cook. Always a healthy eater, her family jokes about her preference for salad over sweets. Since fully taking the plant-based plunge in January 2019, it has been her mission to prove that plants are delicious by creating drool-worthy recipes that make people want to eat their vegetables. In her off time, she enjoys her three small children and laughs at her husband's pranks.

Printed in the USA
CPSIA information can be obtained
at www.ICGtesting.com
JSHW040029010424
59884JS00001B/1